Praise for

Gluten-Free Vegan Comfort Food

"Stuffed with easy to prepare, traditional comfort foods—with the not-so-traditional adjustment of using all gluten-free and vegan ingredients. . . . If you're just starting out on the trail of allergen-free cooking, this book is easy to read and the recipes extremely easy to follow. If you're a pro at this, ingredients will be familiar and you can finally find some recipes for those treasured family favorites!"—*San Francisco Book Review*

"Whether readers are following a gluten-free vegan lifestyle due to medical, health, or ethical reasons, they're likely to find O'Brien's follow-up to *The Gluten-Free Vegan* to be a helpful resource when the craving for comfort food hits. . . . Folks in search of inventive riffs (she's even included a kid-friendly chapter with 'chicken' nuggets that uses tempeh instead of poultry) are sure to find a few new favorites here."—*Publishers Weekly*

"This nifty cookbook proves the point that living a gluten-free lifestyle doesn't mean giving up many of your favorite foods. . . . Complete with information about gluten-free ingredients such as flours and sweeteners, their nutrients, and how they affect a recipe's texture and flavor, this cookbook serves up gluten-free, vegan dishes that are easy and fun to prepare without sacrificing taste. . . . I loved this cookbook."—*Tucson Citizen*

"Recipes, which include things like Mac and Cheese and Chocolate Cupcakes . . . evoke memories of Mom's home cooking. . . . The book includes lists of foods to avoid, pantry essentials and easy-to-understand explanations of unusual ingredients and celiac disease—essential stuff for people who are new to the gluten-free world."—*Portland Oregonian*

Praise for

The Gluten-Free Vegetarian Family Cookbook

"So often, gluten-free and vegetarian processed foods are heavy on sugars, fats, and high-glycemic starches, and low on whole foods. Some GF cookbooks incorporate too many recipes made with unhealthy ingredients. This book is different. It is a great place to start to inspire a gluten-free vegetarian diet that is healthy too! Whether you are just starting out with a GF diet, or have decided to go vegan or vegetarian, or you need some great new recipes to add to your families' menu, this book is for you!"—Sally Johnson, DO, Family Physician

THE GLUTEN-FREE VEGETARIAN
Family Cookbook

ALSO BY Susan O'Brien

Gluten-Free, Sugar-Free Cooking

The Gluten-Free Vegan

Gluten-Free Vegan Comfort Food

THE **GLUTEN-FREE VEGETARIAN**

Family Cookbook

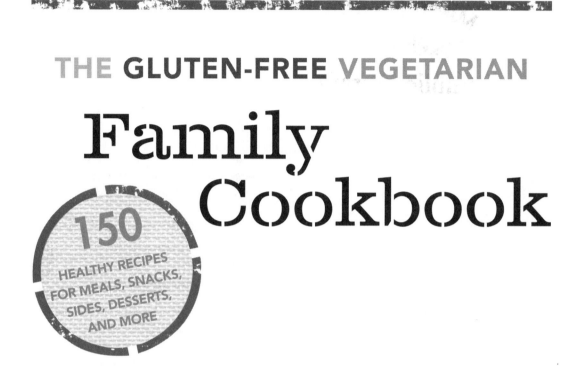

150 HEALTHY RECIPES FOR MEALS, SNACKS, SIDES, DESSERTS, AND MORE

Susan O'Brien

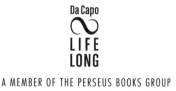

Da Capo
∞
LIFE
LONG

A MEMBER OF THE PERSEUS BOOKS GROUP

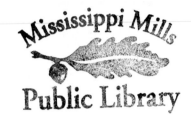

Set in 11 point Warnock Pro Light by the Perseus Books Group

Cataloging-in-Publication data for this book is available from the Library of Congress.

First Da Capo Press edition 2015

LCCN: 2014950432

ISBN: 978-0-7382-1748-2 (paperback)
ISBN: 978-0-7382-1749-9 (ebook)

Published by Da Capo Press
A Member of the Perseus Books Group
www.dacapopress.com

Note: The information in this book is true and complete to the best of our knowledge. This book is intended only as an informative guide for those wishing to know more about health issues. In no way is this book intended to replace, countermand, or conflict with the advice given to you by your own physician. The ultimate decision concerning care should be made between you and your doctor. We strongly recommend you follow his or her advice. Information in this book is general and is offered with no guarantees on the part of the authors or Da Capo Press. The authors and publisher disclaim all liability in connection with the use of this book.

Da Capo Press books are available at special discounts for bulk purchases in the U.S. by corporations, institutions, and other organizations. For more information, please contact the Special Markets Department at the Perseus Books Group, 2300 Chestnut Street, Suite 200, Philadelphia, PA 19103, or call (800) 810-4145, ext. 5000, or e-mail special.markets@perseusbooks.com.

10 9 8 7 6 5 4 3 2 1

THIS BOOK IS DEDICATED TO
MY GRANDCHILDREN,

Nate AND Ella
and in memory of my father,
Stephen J. O'Brien, Jr.

Contents

RECIPES

Breakfast Dishes 17

Breads, Muffins, and Scones 33

Soups and Salads 47

Main Dishes 77

Side Dishes   123

Desserts   147

Snacks, Sauces, Pantry Staples, and Everything Else   171

Foreword

I have known Susan O'Brien for many years, first as a co-worker and then as a friend. Each of her cookbooks has taken me and my patients further along in the quest for healthy eating with special needs, such as gluten-free. Her latest collection of recipes is both family-friendly and gluten-free—a well-needed topic for a cookbook. As I read it through and tried out some recipes, my first thought was: Wow, you did it again, Susan!

I have been eating gluten-free and recommending it to my patients for many years now, and I have been frustrated with the plethora of high-glycemic alternative grains and sweeteners used in most gluten-free foods and recipes. And it can be quite a challenge for kids to accept eating the gluten-free way, especially when siblings or other family members don't eat gluten-free. *The Gluten-Free Vegetarian Family Cookbook* solves those dilemmas: delicious, healthy, appealing recipes . . . with pictures!

You can tell that much research has gone into the development of these creative recipes that avoid the typical high-glycemic gluten-free alternatives. I am excited to try more of the recipes! From chia seeds—the high-fiber, high–omega-3 superfood—to coconut flour or coconut palm sugar . . . and wait until you make your own sauerkraut. Research has shown us that we all need to eat more freshly fermented foods like sauerkraut. And you're in for yet another treat with kelp noodles!

Making your own nut milks? What a concept! It is so easy and cost-effective to make your own, without all the additives that are in the boxed varieties. You'll find some great recipes for nut milks in this cookbook!

Susan has given us comprehensive, up-to-date information on important issues, such as the avoidance of GMO (genetically modified) foods, and stresses the benefits of buying local foods in season. There are a lot of slow cooker recipe books out there, but the ones I have seen use gluten grains and canned foods. While most people are unaware of the health benefits of slow-cooking food, they do know how nice it is to come home to the smell of a home-cooked meal from the slow cooker! This book has it all—up-to-date information and delicious, healthy, gluten-free recipes.

You will be sharing them with your family and friends! I know that I will be recommending this book to my patients, even those who are not gluten-free, because the recipes are delicious. Bon appétit!

Barb Schiltz, RN, MS,
Nutrition Consultant

Introduction

I want to say a big thank you to all of you who have supported my work. Of the cookbooks I've written so far, this one was by far the most fun to create, and I hope you enjoy it as much as I enjoyed creating it for you!

A colleague and friend of mine, Dr. Tom O'Bryan, held The Gluten Summit at the end of 2013. It was a multi-day, online event led by medical experts from around the world. They spoke about why gluten is causing problems for so many people today: Wheat has been modified and is not the same food it was thirty years ago. The protein in wheat, gluten, is difficult to break down in the digestive tract, leaving many of us unable to properly digest it.

The physician experts also talked about other foods that can lead to poor health outcomes. What do you think was at the top of the list? You got it—simple carbohydrates and sugar! Every one of the presenters that I listened to encouraged participants to cut simple carbs out of their diets. A goal well worth considering.

This book focuses on healthy carbs rather than simple carbs, which I'll explain more about further into the book. For that reason, I tried to stay away from sugary desserts and, instead, I am offering ones that include complex carbs and protein. The desserts in this cookbook, if eaten occasionally, are not going to cause you great harm (that is, unless you are a diabetic or have other health conditions that require you to avoid sugar entirely). I believe in moderation, so for your health, dessert should be an occasional treat, not a daily event!

I personally learned a lot during the writing of this book. I used to dislike sauerkraut immensely. Just the smell of it turned me away, but today, I have a crock full of it fermenting on my counter! I have fun creating different variations each time I make a new batch. I hope you will make some yourself, if you haven't already.

Friendly bacteria called *lactobacilli* are formed during the sauerkraut fermentation process. Lactobacilli produce a variety of enzymes that aid digestion and help to increase healthy flora in our digestive tract. I am now eating more sauerkraut and finding unique ways to work it into recipes so that you and your family can benefit from it too.

You will notice that the book includes recipes for vegetarians. There are so many varied diets in our culture today, and even within our own families, so I wanted to offer more options in order to provide a cookbook that would cross the dietary divide. I developed the recipes to be mainly vegan but with many options for those who wish to include dairy products in their diets. You will see that some recipes call for eggs. When it was possible to create the recipe without eggs, I did. I have also provided suggestions for those who wish to add non-dairy cheese to a recipe. I came up with a wonderful "Parmesan" cheese that is made from raw Brazil nuts and a wee bit of garlic and salt. If you are a vegan, you can use this recipe as a cheese alternative, or use your favorite store-bought variety.

I have also made many of the recipes nut-free. Please look carefully at the recipes, as some include substitution ideas for nuts, or I have developed a second recipe that is made with different ingredients. I sincerely hope you find recipes in the book that will not only satisfy your taste buds but also the needs of your family.

For this cookbook, I wanted to focus more on recipes the family would enjoy together, rather than the kids eating one meal and the parents another. When I stopped eating gluten that is exactly how it was in my household. My kids did not "have" to be gluten-free, and they pitched such a fit about it, I ended up making separate meals for all of us. That was nearly twenty years ago, and the gluten-free options were not at all what they are today. Now the entire family can be gluten-free, and they do not have to sacrifice flavor or texture.

The book has icons that show you recipes that are quick and easy to make. You can get dinner to the table quickly and not have to spend an hour fussing with the preparations. These recipes take under thirty minutes to prepare or are cooked slowly throughout the day or during the night while you are sleeping.

I have developed a cookbook with 150 recipes that taste great and are not difficult to prepare. As I say in every book I write, these recipes are a good place to begin. Use your creativity in the kitchen to make foods that you love and that support your own well-being. I wish you all great health. After all, the better care of our bodies we take, the more likely we will live out our lives, fully enjoying each and every day. What else can we ask for?

Kind regards,
Susan

About the Recipes

What's New?

Over the past few years I have come to realize that eating gluten-free (GF) does not necessarily mean eating healthy food. One reason for this is that manufacturers of GF products want to make their products taste good so they will sell; as a result, these products often contain lots of fat, salt, and sugar. Another reason is many GF people complain that GF products do not have the same "lift" or lightness that products made with gluten have. This is true, as gluten provides structure to baked goods, and its elasticity and chewiness is hard to reproduce in gluten-free products! Unfortunately, many gluten-free baked goods are not very good for you, as they are high in starch or simple carbs, which are used to replicate the texture of gluten-containing foods. For example, potato starch, cornstarch, and tapioca starch are all used in many GF foods to improve the texture and to provide lightness. Tapioca starch is high in carbohydrates (30 percent of your daily allotted value in just 3.53 ounces) and has no health benefits. Cornstarch is made from genetically modified corn, so I don't recommend it in my recipes. I do use arrowroot powder in a few of the recipes in the book, as it is helps to thicken sauces.

Simple carbs are found in foods such as cereals, breads, pasta, potato chips, fruit, candy, honey, soda, and jam. Some simple sugars, such as fruit, are not bad for you, but you want to eat them in moderation. Most simple carbs provide very little nutritional value and are made up of one or two sugars. Due to their simple nature, they are processed by the body very quickly. This is why if you eat a doughnut for breakfast, you are hungry again in an hour!

Complex carbs, on the other hand, are made up of three or four sugars that are often linked up to form a chain. Complex carbs are full of fiber, vitamins, and minerals and are found in vegetables, whole grains, and foods made with them. They are processed slower by the body and take

3

longer to digest, which is why you feel fuller longer when you eat a bowl of amaranth for breakfast instead of that doughnut. Complex carbohydrates fuel the body. They give us energy, and they don't raise blood sugar as rapidly as simple sugars and carbohydrates.

Complex carbs offer a higher nutritional value than simple carbs, and for that reason, I have done my best to focus on utilization of complex carbs in this cookbook. Simple carbs should be avoided, if possible, especially for those with diabetes or those, like myself, who are always striving to improve my diet and overall well-being. I have embarked down an exciting path that focuses more on complex carbs and less on simple carbs. You will see teff, almond meal and flour, buckwheat, coconut, and sorghum flours used in this book in the desserts, breads, and muffins sections. Have no fear! The recipes are delicious, and they are better for you, as they offer more protein and other nutrients, so you can feel good about serving them to your family.

The recipes in this book also offer a variety of sources of protein. I grew up being told that the best source of protein was meat and dairy. I believed what I was told, and I ate meat and dairy. Oddly enough, my body didn't do well with either of those foods, and I often had digestive issues. Today, many years later, I know that I can get protein from a whole host of foods, including, but not limited to: beans, lentils, legumes, seeds, nuts, and whole grains, as well as vegetables, and yes, believe it or not, even fruits! Dried apricots contain the highest amount of protein in a fruit, offering 5 percent protein in a half cup of fruit. Dried prunes and currants come in at 4 percent, and berries clock in at a mere 1 percent per half cup, but that is better than nothing! One medium sweet potato contains about 2 grams of protein, and one large stalk of broccoli sports about 4 grams of protein. While it is difficult to get all of your protein needs from vegetables and fruits, you certainly can add nuts, seeds, legumes, and other foods to round out your protein intake.

When you make these recipes, I highly recommend you seek out foods that are organic and not genetically modified. To genetically modify an organism, scientists utilize a process to alter their genes with DNA from other species of living organisms to achieve "desired traits" like tolerance to pesticides and resistance to disease. Genetically modified foods (commonly referred to as GMO foods) are now on about 60–70 percent of the US grocery store shelves. Most processed foods contain GMOs, which is why I recommend you stay away from them! Not only are processed foods high in simple carbs, they also are made with GMO ingredients like soy and corn.

While there is a need for more research into why GMO foods are not good for our health, a French study, which was published in the *International Journal of Biosciences* in 2009, showed that toxicity increased in rats fed GMO corn, and the organs most affected were the kidney and liver, but also the heart, adrenal glands, spleen, and haematopoietic system.[*]

GMO foods also have adverse effects on the environment. Most GM crops are engineered to be "herbicide tolerant." Roundup ready crops, sold by Monsanto, for example, are designed to survive multiple applications of the herbicide called Roundup. According to the Institute for Responsible Technology, US farmers sprayed 383 million pounds of herbicides on GM foods between 1996 and 2008. The bad news is that overuse of Roundup results in plants that are resistant to herbicides, and these foods end up containing higher residues of the pesticides, which are toxic, especially those with Roundup. Eating these foods has been linked to hormone disruption, birth defects, and cancer.

In the Resources section of this book, I have provided some suggested reading for you regarding GMOs. I hope you take a moment to read this information, as it may help you make better selections the next time you go to the market.

------

[*] Joël Spiroux de Vendômois, François Roullier, Dominique Cellier, and Gilles-Éric Séralini, "A Comparison of the Effects of Three GM Corn Varieties on Mammalian Health," *International Journal of Biological Sciences* 5, no. 7 (2009): 706–726, DOI:10.7150/ijbs.5.706, http://www.ijbs .com/v05p0706.htm.

If a food is labeled organic, it cannot be genetically modified. Remember this when you are out shopping! I also am very conscious of how much GF, GMO-free, organic foods can cost, so in the last recipe chapter (Snacks, Sauces, Pantry Staples, and Everything Else, page 171), I added recipes that teach you how to make your own nut milks, almond butter, almond meal, sauerkraut, non-dairy cheese, and more.

What Is Sustainable Eating? Healthier Food for People and the Planet

Eating sustainable is not difficult. There are benefits to our bodies and our planet when we embark on a sustainable lifestyle. I say lifestyle instead of diet because to be sustainable, we need to make some behavior changes too. What follows are some ideas that will help you live a more sustainable lifestyle.

Eat organic. Sustainable food tastes better because it is grown locally, and it is usually organic and grown without pesticides. Locally grown organic fruits and vegetables are also GMO-free, so they are better for your health!

Eat foods in season, shop at farmers' markets or local markets rather than large grocery store chains, and grow your own food whenever you can. Grow a container garden on your back porch!

Consider canning the foods you grow or buy at local farmers' markets. It is very satisfying to make your own tomato sauce, salsa, ketchup, and jams. I used to make all of my own for my young family, and I loved seeing the kitchen cabinets full of organic foods that I put up myself. It is rewarding, and the best benefit is that you know what your family is eating.

Buying in bulk is better for the environment, as there are fewer containers that get thrown away, filling up the landfills. Buying in bulk is more economical and usually the foods are fresher because the high turnaround means less time spent on the shelf. Say good-bye to plastic if you can too.

Bring your own bags to the market to help reduce waste.

Consider participating in a community garden with your family. It's a fun way to teach the kids how to grow food, and it's a great way to eat well and ensure your crops are not sprayed with pesticides. Or, grow your own garden! I don't have the yard space anymore for one, so I have a container garden on my deck. Kids love to watch things grow, and it sure is nice to have those herbs right outside the door all summer long.

Shop at or join a food co-op. Often group discounts are provided. Co-ops work hard to establish good relationships with local farmers, so you know where the food comes from.

Buy Fair Trade products, as they are economically fair and environmentally sustainable. In this ever-changing world, we need to be mindful of our carbon footprint on the planet. Look for the Fair Trade symbol when shopping for coffee, tea, chocolate, and other products.

Become aware of the "Dirty Dozen" (foods that you only want to eat organic). They include: apples, strawberries, grapes, celery, cherry tomatoes, cucumbers, nectarines, peaches, potatoes, kale/chard, sweet bell peppers, and summer squash.

Check out the Environmental Working Group website for the "Clean Fifteen" and more: http://www.ewg.org/foodnews /summary.php.

Eating foods in season is not something many of us think about. At the store, we see a fruit or vegetable we want, and we put it into our carts. I encourage you to check the label to find out where that product came from. If you are buying watermelon in New York in the winter, it is very unlikely that watermelon was grown anywhere nearby. Try to eat foods that are in season when you're buying them. For instance, in the spring, peas and asparagus are so crisp and delicious; in the winter, acorn squash and yams are at their peak! Go on a journey with your kids to find out what foods are grown locally throughout the year and then find new ways to cook with those foods. I think you will have fun and learn a lot! Check out the Resources section for some great websites to learn more.

In every book I write, I share products that I like, and I have some new favorites! Check out my must-haves.

Kelp noodles: They are a great alternative to rice pasta. I always keep these noodles stocked in my refrigerator so I can quickly make a stir-fry with them or toss them in a salad or soup. You do not have to cook kelp noodles; they are ready to eat once you rinse them and cut into bite-size pieces. Sea Tangle brand kelp noodles are low in carbs and calories, and they are fat-free and allergen-free. A 4-ounce serving contains only 6 calories and 1 gram of carbohydrate. You can buy them at local stores, such as Whole Foods, Mother's Market, food co-ops, Cream of the Crop, Asian markets, and Papaya's Natural Foods, or you can find them on Amazon. Or buy them online at www.kelpnoodles.com.

Tofu shirataki noodles, such as House Foods brand, are a great spaghetti noodle substitute that is GMO-free, GF, and vegan, with only 20 calories per serving and 3 grams of carbs. They are delicious in soups! This noodle is made from the flour of the *konjac*—an Asian yam—and tofu. Look for shirataki noodles in Asian groceries and health-food stores, or online at www.house-foods.com.

Coconut oil (organic): Coconut oil stays solid when cold, softens like butter at room temperature, and melts when heated. A note about coconut oil: It is good to know that if you live in a warm climate, or you have hot summers, coconut oil will turn to liquid once it reaches 76°F. I do not recommend

keeping it in the refrigerator, but if you go to the cupboard one day and find it in its liquid form, don't worry, it is fine; when it cools down, it will return to a solid state. I like Carrington Farms brand coconut oil, as it is certified organic and contains no trans or hydrogenated fats. It's unrefined, cold-pressed, 100 percent extra virgin coconut oil. I use mostly coconut and olive oil in this book, but occasionally I use sesame seed oil and grapeseed oil. If you are interested in learning where you can buy Carrington Farms coconut oil, go to www.carringtonfarms.com.

Coconut cream: I use coconut cream in several of the recipes in this cookbook. There are different types of coconut cream on the market, including those sold at Trader Joe's and health-food stores. Depending on your preference, budget, and proximity to a market that carries coconut cream, you have many options to choose from. Kara is one brand that I have used, but it is not organic. If you wish to stay with organic, you might consider Tropical Traditions brand (www.tropicaltraditions.com) or Native Forest unsweetened coconut cream (www.edwardandsons.com), which is certified GMO-free and organic.

Coconut milk (dairy replacement): Many companies are now producing coconut milk. I use it in my morning latte and for baking. If you want to stay organic, I would recommend So Delicious coconut milk.

Silk brand coconut milk is certified non-GMO, but it is not organic; Trader Joe's brand coconut milk also is not organic.

Coconut milk (concentrate): There are several organic options for concentrated coconut milk. I recommend Native Forest, Edward and Sons, or Thai Kitchen. I use canned coconut milk in curries, puddings, or soups to replace milk or cream.

Helen's Kitchen Organic Veggie Ground and Chorizo: These vegetable-based meat substitutes are GMO-free and organic. One serving is 2 ounces and provides 60 calories, 3.5 grams of which are from fat. There are a total of 5 grams of carbohydrates and 5 grams of protein. Visit their website to learn where you can find the products and read a list of their ingredients: www.the helenskitchen.com.

Tofu, tempeh, and miso: I used tofu or fermented soy in several of the recipes in this book. There has been a lot of research conducted over the years about the risks and benefits of soy in the diet. I have listed some links in the References section of the book that will provide more information on the health benefits and concerns of soy. I personally only buy non-GMO organic tofu, and I hope you will do the same, as many other soy products have been genetically modified. In my humble opinion, genetically modified foods are NOT good for us, mainly because of the effects on the environment and the possible impacts on our health. A very well-respected functional medicine physician, Dr. Mark Hyman, provides his take on the soy controversy on his blog.[*] He says if you want to reduce your risk for breast cancer, stop eating trans fats and drink less alcohol—soy is not the culprit. Dr. Hyman says to consume whole soy rather than processed soy. I use tempeh, miso, and edamame in this cookbook because I agree wholeheartedly that soy is not bad for us if we are not allergic to it and we eat whole or fermented soy.

If you are allergic to soy, or have had a history of breast cancer, you may want to substitute other ingredients for the soy listed in the recipes. If substituting with legumes or another protein source is not possible, then I would recommend that you skip the recipe and find another that better suits your dietary needs. (Note that many of these recipes are already soy-free!)

Please be aware that not all tempeh and miso are gluten-free. Some miso is made with barley, so make sure you read the label to ensure it is made with rice. Some tempeh contains added soy sauce, so read the label to be sure it is truly GF.

---

[*]Mark Hyman, "How Soy Can Kill You and Save Your Life," DrHyman.com, August 6, 2010, http://drhyman.com/blog/2010/08/06/how-soy-can-kill-you-and-save-your-life.

Chia seeds: Oh, chia seeds! I love them and they are so good for us! These little seeds are a powerhouse of protein (20 percent of your daily value) and alanine amino acid (20 percent of your daily value), and are very high in omega-3 fatty acids, fiber, calcium, iron, and vitamin C. I have been using chia seeds as an egg replacer for years now, and I love how well they mimic the consistency of an egg. If you are a vegan, you will want to substitute the eggs in the baked goods recipes in this book—consider using chia seeds! For every egg in a recipe, place 1 teaspoon of chia seeds in a small bowl and add 2 tablespoons of water. Whisk them together well, then set the mixture aside to gel. In about 5 minutes, stir the mixture again and then it is ready to use.

Sprouts: I love growing my own sprouts. I ordered a sprout contraption about two years ago, and now I always have fresh sprouts in the house. Mung beans are my favorite to spout, but I also like quinoa, broccoli, millet, alfalfa, sunflower seeds, and more! Sprouts contain up to a hundred times more enzymes than uncooked veggies and fruits. They are also high in vitamins A, B, and C. And they are a good source of fiber and essential fatty acids.

Quinoa: By now most people know what quinoa is (pronounced *keen-wah*), but do you know how good it is for you? Quinoa isn't really a "true grain"—it's a plant that is related to both chard and spinach. It is super high in protein (contains nine essential amino acids) and is also high in fiber. One cup of cooked quinoa contains 3.6 grams of fat, 5.2 grams of fiber, and 8 grams of protein, with a total of 222 calories. I use quinoa in soups, stews, and stuffed squash, and in place of rice in pilafs, salads, and other dishes. It is very versatile and has a sweet nutty flavor.

Cinnamon: I love the flavor of cinnamon and use it all the time. I have included it in many of the recipes in this book. You may wonder why I am talking about a spice in this section of the book, but cinnamon has amazing health benefits. Researchers at the National Center for Biotechnology Information found that consuming cinnamon every day could improve cholesterol and glucose levels. Their study followed sixty adults with Type 2 diabetes. The participants were asked to consume 1–6 grams of cinnamon per day for forty days. Those who followed through with the requirement reduced their glucose levels by 18–29 percent and reduced their bad cholesterol (LDL) by 6–27 percent.

Mochi: Mochi is a traditional Japanese food that is made from sweet short-grain rice. It is all-natural, made without preservatives or additives, and can be used in a variety of ways.

Mochi is gluten- and dairy-free. There are many varieties to choose from, and they come in different flavors, such as raisin and cinnamon, sesame and garlic, pizza flavor, or my favorite, super seed mochi (made with organic sweet brown rice, hemp seeds, pumpkin seeds, flax seeds, sesame seeds, poppy seeds, and sunflower seeds). The brand I like is Grainaissance, but you can also make your own mochi—search online for instructional videos on how to make it.

Most often, mochi is made into a snack. I do not prepare mochi the traditional way, which is to steam or pan-fry it; instead, I bake it in the oven or cook it in a waffle iron (see my recipe for Mochi Waffles on page 23). To bake this snack in the oven, simply cut the square slab of mochi into 1½-inch squares and place them on a baking sheet. Bake them in an oven that has been pre-heated to 450°F for 8–10 minutes. They will puff up during the baking process. You can find many mochi recipes online or on the back of the package too.

Sauerkraut: I have fallen in love with sauerkraut. I make my own fresh sauerkraut every month and eat it every day. Why? Because it is GOOD for us! As sauerkraut ferments, friendly *lactobacilli* and enzymes are created that help with digestion and keep our intestinal flora healthy. Cabbage is high in vitamins A and C. It is also a rich source of phytonutrients. I make my sauerkraut out of green cabbage. I also like to add carrots and apples, but you do not

have to add anything but cabbage if you don't want to! Check out the recipes for homemade sauerkraut on pages 188 and 190 in this book.

Bragg's Amino Acids: Amino acids are the building blocks of our tissues and organs. Sometimes our bodies do not produce enough amino acids to break down and properly digest the foods we eat, so we miss out on important nutrients and minerals that our bodies need. Adding amino acids to recipes in place of tamari reduces the sodium level and adds the essential acids our bodies need. Essential amino acids in Bragg's include: arginine, aspartic, lysine, glutamic, serine, threonine, alanine, glycine, proline, isoleucine, methionine, valine, phenylalanine, tyrosine, and leucine. Bragg's uses non-GMO soybeans to make all of their products. Find out more at www.bragg.com.

Organic coconut palm sugar: Use coconut palm sugar as you would regular sugar (one to one) for sweetness without the highs and lows in your blood sugar. I like Big Tree Farms brand, which is unrefined, vegan, and non-GMO. It is pure coconut flower blossom nectar that is low glycemic and high in nutrients, and it has sixteen amino acids. Check out their website and list of where to buy it in your neighborhood: http://bigtreefarms.com.

Flours and Other Pantry Staples

Flours

I recommend using **Whole-Grain Flours** in your recipes whenever possible. What are whole grains? Whole grains include 100 percent of the original kernel from the seed, such as the germ, bran, and endosperm. Celiacs and those with a gluten sensitivity must use gluten-free flours. There are many on the market today. Gluten-free whole-grain flours include: amaranth, buckwheat, millet, quinoa, oat, brown rice, sorghum, and teff. I use the following flours in this book.

ALMOND MEAL OR FLOUR

I love using almond meal or flour in baked goods because of its nutritional contributions (¼ cup provides 6 grams of protein, 3 grams of fiber, and 1 gram of sugar, and it is high in magnesium and vitamin E). You can make your own almond meal or flour (see the last recipe chapter [Snacks, Sauces, Pantry Staples, and Everything Else], page 171). Storing this flour or meal in the refrigerator will extend its freshness and prevent rancidity.

BROWN RICE FLOUR

Brown rice flour is not as healthy of a flour as the others, but it is a good source of fiber, vitamin B, and iron. Because brown rice flour is processed with the kernel intact, it contains more oil than white rice flour. For this reason, it can go rancid quickly, and I recommend storing it in the refrigerator.

BUCKWHEAT FLOUR

The name buckwheat really throws some people for a loop. It's not a member of the wheat family at all; it hails from the rhubarb and sorrel families. Buckwheat provides B1, B2, magnesium, phosphate, potassium, and more iron than cereal grains.

COCONUT FLOUR

Coconut flour adds protein, fiber (2 tablespoons provides 5 grams of fiber and 8 grams of carbs), calcium, and flavor to a recipe. Organic coconut flour is easily found in health-food stores and online. It can be expensive, so if you want to make your own, use organic flaked raw, unsweetened coconut and whirl it in a food processor until it is fine like flour. I never use this flour alone, as it is very dense, so be sure to use it in combination with other flours, like brown rice, sorghum, or almond (up to 20 percent of the total flour). I recommend storing it in the refrigerator or freezer to maintain its freshness.

GARBANZO BEAN FLOUR

Garbanzos, also called chickpeas, are a legume that is high in protein (6 grams of protein per quarter cup) and fiber (5 grams per quarter cup), with only 2 grams of fat (per quarter cup) and 18 grams of carbohydrate (3 gram from sugar). Garbanzo beans provide phytonutrients and also provide calcium, iron, and vitamin C.

SORGHUM FLOUR

Sorghum flour is great as a replacement for wheat flour because it seems to mimic the texture the best, it is not grainy like rice flours, and it has a little bit of a nutty flavor. One cup of sorghum flour provides 9.5 grams of protein, 8 grams of fiber, and 2.3 grams of sugar. I store all of my flours in the vegetable bins in the refrigerator to preserve their freshness.

TEFF FLOUR

This tiny grain (smallest in the world) is a powerhouse of nutrition! A quarter cup contains 4 grams of protein, 4 grams of fiber, and zero sugar. It is high in iron, amino acids, vitamin C, and calcium. If you want the kids to eat foods made with teff, only use teff flour for about a quarter of the total flour in a recipe, as the flavor can be a bit overwhelming—not in a bad way, but it is a heavier flour that has its own unique flavor.

These flours are readily available in markets around the country, but if you live in a rural area where it is hard to find these flours, I would recommend that you shop online. Today you can even buy flour from Amazon! The following companies offer great GF flours:

King Arthur Flour: www.kingarthurflour.com
Bob's Red Mill: www.bobsredmill.com
Namaste Foods: www.namastefoods.com
Arrowhead Mills: www.arrowheadmills.com

Also check out www.celiaccentral.org for more information on GF suppliers and manufacturers.

Gluten-Free Oats and Oat Flour

Many companies have come out with certified gluten-free oats. This is great news for those with celiac disease, but many people still worry that oats are not safe to eat. According to the Celiac Support Association, certified GF oats may be safe for many people but not all. Avenin, a protein found in oats, is very similar to gluten and can cause an adverse reaction in some people. If you are a celiac, medical experts advise that you should not introduce gluten-free oats into your diet until your symptoms resolve, and then, add them in slowly to ensure you do not have a reaction. Please check with your doctor before introducing oats into your diet.

I make my own oat flour from certified gluten-free oats. If you have celiac disease and you have determined that oats are safe for you, I recommend that you make your own oat flour too. This will ensure you do not have an adverse reaction, as the oat flours on the market are not, as far as I know, certified GF. To make oat flour, simply put the oats in a food processor and whirl until fine. Make only the amount that your recipe calls for. I don't make oat flour in advance or store it, I only make it as needed in recipes, so it does not turn rancid.

Baking Powder

Some varieties of baking powder are NOT gluten-free, so be sure to read the labels before you buy it. You can also make your own baking powder by combining the following:

¼ cup baking soda

½ cup cream of tartar

½ cup arrowroot powder

Stir this mixture together well and store it in a glass jar in your pantry or in some other cool, dry location.

Guar Gum

This thickener is the endosperm of the guar bean. It is typically grown in Australia and India. It is used to thicken foods and act as a stabilizer. I use it occasionally in baked goods.

Arrowroot Powder

Arrowroot is a plant typically grown in the Caribbean or in a similar climate. Arrowroot powder is a highly digestible starch that is used primarily as a thickener for sauces, soups, puddings, etc.

Sweeteners

In this book, I primarily use brown rice syrup, organic maple syrup, or organic coconut palm sugar. If you wish to avoid sugar in any form, you might want to ex-periment with stevia. I do not use stevia in this cookbook, but there are many books on the market that use stevia, and they provide guidance on how to modify recipes. Because I rarely eat desserts or sugar in general, I went with the products that would produce the best outcome without being overly sweet. I balanced the sugars with protein-rich flours in an attempt to make desserts that could be appreciated and enjoyed by the entire family. Just remember, whether you're using coconut palm sugar, brown rice syrup, maple syrup, or honey, sugar is sugar, no matter how you slice it. So I stand by the philosophy "all things in moderation!"

BROWN RICE SYRUP

Lundberg Brown Rice Syrup is organic, gluten-free, kosher, and vegan, and 2 tablespoons equals 22 grams of sugar, or 150 calories.

ORGANIC MAPLE SYRUP

Researchers from the University of Rhode Island have found that maple syrup from Canada is filled with anti-inflammatory and antioxidant compounds that may have health benefits, such as helping diabetics keep their blood sugars balanced. There are 104 calories in 2 tablespoons of maple syrup and 23 grams of sugar.[*]

---

[*] "Maple Syrup's Health Benefits," Health News Report, April 2, 2011, http://healthnewsreport .blogspot.com/2011/04/maple-syrups-health -benefits.html.

HONEY

Honey has a long medicinal history and many people believe it has strong anti-bacterial and anti-inflammatory proper-ties. The darker the color of the honey, the higher its antioxidant power, according to some studies. Never give honey to children under the age of one. One tablespoon of honey provides about 60 calories and 16 grams of sugar.

Alcohol

Some of the recipes in this book call for a touch of wine. Distilled alcoholic bever-ages are gluten-free with the exception of beer, ales, and lagers. Many companies are now producing gluten-free beers. Wine and hard liquor are also gluten-free, even though there are many people who believe otherwise. If you drink wine coolers or fla-vored wine, there is no guarantee it is 100 percent gluten-free, but wine made from 100 percent grapes is GF. Wine is not made with grains like beer. The stats I found in-dicate that wine is gluten-free to 20 parts per million or less.

The caution about wine or beer is the same as the caution about carbs. Alcohol is high in sugar, and sugar, as we know, is not good for us. So, again, my mantra . . . everything in moderation!

The Gluten-Free Vegetarian Pantry: Foods to Stock

I have listed items I recommend for sup-porting a healthy gluten-free vegetarian diet. You may have more, but this is a good place to start!

Flours

Almond flour

Buckwheat flour

Teff flour

Coconut flour

Sorghum four

Brown rice flour

Garbanzo bean (chickpea) flour

Quinoa flour

Millet flour

Amaranth flour

Bob's Red Mills Gluten-Free All Purpose Flour

Organic cornmeal

Other Dry Ingredients

Chia seeds

Flax seeds

Almond meal

GF oats

Nutritional yeast

Arrowroot

Cornmeal

Sweeteners

Organic maple syrup

Organic brown rice syrup

Organic coconut palm sugar

Pure fruit jams

Organic applesauce

Molasses

Raw honey

Oils and Other Fats

Coconut oil, virgin and organic

Olive oil, cold-pressed and extra virgin

Grapeseed oil, expeller or cold-pressed

Roasted sesame oil

Spectrum organic palm shortening

Earth Balance non-GMO spread

Ghee

Coconut and olive oil spray

Standard Staples

Brown rice

Red rice

Arborio rice

Wild rice

Black rice

Quinoa

Lentils

Mung beans

Dried beans

Rice noodles

Seaweed

Dried peas and seeds

Nuts and seeds

Raisins, Medjool dates, dried cherries and cranberries

Balsamic vinegar

Apple cider vinegar (I prefer Bragg's brand)

Brown rice vinegar

Rice vinegar

GF tamari sauce

GF teriyaki sauce

Nut and seed butters

Organic vegetable broth

Vanilla extract

Vegan chocolate chips (I prefer Enjoy Life brand)

Peppercorns

Fresh and dried herbs

Spices

Candied ginger

Cocoa powder

Baking yeast

Guar gum

Baking soda

GF baking powder

Himalayan salt, kosher salt, sea salt

Kelp flakes

Red and white wine

Breakfast
Dishes

Best Sunrise Breakfast Muffins

These muffins are great to have with your favorite morning beverage or to serve alongside a veggie scramble. Almond meal adds protein, and apple and carrots provide fiber and the energy to get up and go! If you are allergic to nuts, you can substitute sorghum flour for the almond meal or flour and use sunflower seeds in place of the walnuts. I have a huge muffin pan, so I make about nine BIG muffins at a time, but if you have a standard muffin pan, this recipe makes twelve muffins.

MAKES 12 MUFFINS • PREP TIME: 45 MINUTES

¼ cup coconut oil

¼ cup organic unsweetened applesauce

¾ cup coconut palm sugar (or ½ cup sugar and ¼ cup brown sugar)

2 eggs, beaten

1 teaspoon vanilla extract

¼ cup coconut milk (not canned) or water

½ cup sorghum flour

1½ cups almond meal or flour

1 teaspoon baking soda

2 teaspoons baking powder

1 teaspoon guar gum

2 teaspoons cinnamon

½ teaspoon sea salt

1 cup GF oats

1 cup grated apple

1 cup grated carrot

½ cup pitted and chopped Medjool dates (or raisins)

½ cup finely chopped walnuts (or sunflower seeds)

1. Preheat the oven to 350°F. Lightly grease a muffin tin with coconut oil or line the cups with paper muffin liners.

2. In a large mixing bowl, combine the coconut oil, applesauce, and sugar. Beat until light and fluffy. Add in the eggs, vanilla extract, and coconut milk, and stir to blend well. Add in the sorghum flour, almond meal, baking soda, baking powder, guar gum, cinnamon, and salt, and stir on medium-high to fully incorporate. Add in the oats, apple, carrot, dates, and walnuts, and stir together well.

3. Add a ladleful of batter to each muffin cup (fill each about halfway full). Bake for approximately 30 minutes, or until a toothpick inserted in the center comes out clean. Cool on a wire rack.

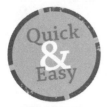

Coconut and
Blueberry Pancakes

Get your morning going with these protein-packed pancakes! Not only are they good for you, they also taste great. Even fussy eaters will enjoy this recipe! Coconut tends to burn easily, so cook these pancakes on a lower temperature than you would normal pancakes. I cook these over medium heat, not medium-high.

SERVES 4 • PREP TIME: ABOUT 5 MINUTES TO PREPARE AND 20 MINUTES TO COOK

½ cup coconut flour

½ cup sorghum flour or brown rice flour

1 teaspoon baking powder

½ teaspoon cinnamon

¼ teaspoon sea salt

1 teaspoon chia seeds

2 tablespoons water

1 egg, beaten

2¼ cups coconut milk (not canned) or other milk of your choosing

1 teaspoon vanilla extract

2 tablespoons coconut oil, melted

½ cup blueberries or other berry

Coconut oil spray for the skillet

1. Mix the coconut flour, sorghum or brown rice flour, baking powder, cinnamon, and salt together in a large bowl.

2. In a smaller bowl, whisk the chia seeds with the water and set aside for 5 minutes to let the mixture gel.

3. Add the egg, milk, vanilla extract, and oil to the chia seed mixture and stir together to blend. Add the liquid ingredients to the dry ingredients and stir to combine. Fold in the berries.

4. Heat a large skillet over medium heat and lightly spray it with coconut oil. When the skillet is hot, add a ladleful of the pancake batter. (If your batter is too thick, add a small amount of water or milk to thin it down to the consistency you prefer.) Cook until bubbles appear in the center, then flip and continue to cook until done. Serve with your favorite topping.

Note: This recipe makes a lot of pancakes. I store any leftover batter in an airtight Tupperware container in the refrigerator. The batter will last up to a week. Thin with additional milk if needed.

Delightful Teff Waffles

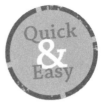

These power-packed waffles are a great start to the day. They are tasty, full of protein and complex carbs, and a snap to make! Serve them with jam, yogurt, applesauce, nut or seed butter, or plain. These waffles freeze well and can be reheated in a toaster for an afternoon snack or for traveling in the car. They will keep frozen for a few months, if they last that long without being eaten!

MAKES 8 TO 10 WAFFLES ◆ **PREP TIME: ABOUT 30 MINUTES, PLUS COOKING TIME**

2 eggs and 2 teaspoons chia seeds whisked with 4 tablespoons water (or 4 eggs)

1 tablespoon vanilla extract

¾ cup milk (or non-dairy milk of your choice; I used coconut milk)

3 tablespoons coconut oil, melted

2 tablespoons honey, molasses, or maple syrup

1½ cups teff flour

3 teaspoons baking powder

¼ teaspoon sea salt

1 teaspoon cinnamon

¼ cup berries (optional)

1. Combine the chia seeds and water in a large bowl and whisk together well. Set aside for 4–5 minutes so the mixture can gel.

2. Add the two eggs, vanilla extract, and milk to the chia mixture and beat well. (If you're not using the chia seeds, add the four eggs, vanilla extract, and milk in a large bowl and beat well.)

3. Stir in the melted coconut oil and the honey (or molasses or maple syrup) and mix well. (If you use honey, it may help to heat it together with the oil in a small saucepan over medium heat and stir so it dissolves a bit.)

4. Add the teff flour, baking powder, sea salt, and cinnamon. Stir to fully blend the wet and dry ingredients. If desired, add the berries and fold them into the batter.

5. Heat a waffle iron and cook the batter according to the manufacturer's directions. Serve immediately; freeze any leftovers.

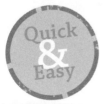

Yam and Banana Waffles

If you have a yam lying around and you don't know what to do with just one yam, this recipe answers that question! You can also use one cup of canned pumpkin purée. There is no need to add sweeteners to this recipe if you are using really ripe bananas! These waffles are tasty and filled with good nutrients, and they are a great way to start your day. I recommend cooking the entire batch at one time, then freezing the waffles, so you can pull one out at a moment's notice and pop it into the toaster. They are a great afternoon snack or quick mid-morning pick-me-up. I am not making any recommendations for toppings, as I don't think they need any, but if desired, top the waffles with your favorite accoutrements.

MAKES 12 WAFFLES ◆ PREP TIME: 10 MINUTES TO PREPARE, PLUS COOKING TIME

1 cup cooked, mashed yams

1 large ripe banana, mashed (about ½ cup)

½ cup milk (coconut, hemp, cashew, or dairy)

4 eggs, beaten well

1 tablespoon coconut oil

½ teaspoon vanilla extract

1 cup coconut cream

1 cup sorghum flour

1½ tablespoons coconut flour or unsweetened finely shredded coconut (optional)

2 tablespoons almond meal (or 2 tablespoons additional sorghum flour)

2 teaspoons baking powder

½ teaspoon cinnamon

¼–½ teaspoon dried ginger

Pinch of sea salt

1. In a large bowl, mash the yams and banana together.

2. Add the milk, beaten eggs, coconut oil, vanilla extract, and coconut cream and beat together well. Add the flours, baking powder, cinnamon, ginger, and salt and whisk well.

3. Heat a waffle iron and cook the batter according to the manufacturer's directions. Serve immediately; freeze any leftovers.

Mochi Waffles

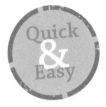

Mochi is made from short-grain sweet rice. It is not a complex carb by itself, but the variety that I like the best is made with hemp seeds, pumpkin seeds, flax seeds, sesame seeds, poppy seeds, and sunflower seeds, which adds greatly to its nutritional value. You can eat these waffles by themselves, or top them with nut or seed butter, hummus, avocado and sprouts, all-fruit jam, or eggs! I also like to take these along in the car to munch on or have as a snack while working.

MAKES 8 WAFFLES ◆ PREP TIME: 3 MINUTES TO PREPARE, PLUS COOKING TIME

1 (12.5-ounce) package mochi (flavor of your choosing)

1. Lay the square slab of mochi on a cutting board and cut in half, crosswise. Then cut in half again, lengthwise, so that you end up with four squares, about 2 × 2 inches. Cut each square in half, from top to bottom (do this carefully, as the mochi is thin and you don't want to slice it too thin). You will end up with eight squares.

2. Heat your waffle iron and when the "ready" light comes on, place two squares of mochi in the waffle iron and cook until the "ready" light reappears. The mochi will have puffed up and is ready to eat. If your waffle iron isn't hot enough, the mochi will not rise and may not be cooked enough. It should be crispy on the outside and chewy on the inside. Continue this process, cooking two squares at a time, until you have eight puffed waffles. Serve immediately.

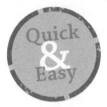

Oats and
Apple Griddlecakes

These are not your traditional pancakes by any stretch of the imagination! They are quite simple to make, and because they are made with chia seeds, they are high in protein and fiber! I have added a small amount of tofu to increase the protein and to add some creaminess to the griddlecakes, but you can leave it out if you prefer. Top the cakes with your choice of toppings, such as fruit, yogurt, or applesauce, or eat them just as they are!

MAKES ABOUT 10 TO 12 GRIDDLECAKES • PREP TIME: ABOUT 30 MINUTES

1 tablespoon chia seeds

1½ cups milk (coconut, hemp, almond, soy, or dairy)

1 teaspoon vanilla extract

1 tablespoon organic maple syrup or brown rice syrup

1½ ounces tofu, puréed (about 3 tablespoons) (optional)

1 large crisp apple, grated (about 1 cup)

1 egg, beaten (optional)

1½ cups organic, GF oats (not quick cooking)

2 teaspoons baking powder

1 teaspoon cinnamon

¼ teaspoon sea salt

Coconut oil spray for the skillet

1. Place the chia seeds and milk in a large bowl and whisk together. Let sit for about 5 minutes to allow it to gel.

2. Add the vanilla extract, maple syrup, puréed tofu, grated apple, and egg (if using) and stir well. Next, add the oats, baking powder, cinnamon, and salt. Stir well to fully incorporate the wet and dry ingredients. Set this mixture aside for 10–15 minutes to allow the oats to soften and the mixture to thicken.

3. Heat a small skillet or griddle over medium heat and lightly spray the pan with coconut oil. When the skillet is hot, add ¼ cup of the batter to the skillet or griddle and cook until bubbles begin to appear around the edges, 2–3 minutes. Flip and cook on the other side for another 2–2½ minutes, or until golden brown. Continue this process until all of the griddlecakes are cooked.

Note: If you prefer not to use all the batter, you can store the leftover batter in an airtight container in the refrigerator. The batter will last for a few days. To reuse the batter, thin it out with milk and repeat the cooking process.

Potato and Zucchini Pancakes

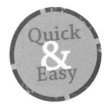

This is a hearty meal to get your day going! This can be served for breakfast, at a Sunday brunch, or as a healthy afternoon snack. I use Herbes de Provence in this dish, but you can substitute Italian seasonings, such as oregano, rosemary, and basil, or a blend of these herbs, or just use salt and fresh cracked pepper. If you want to spice up the recipe a bit, consider adding pinches of cumin, chili powder, and cayenne pepper. That will really fire up your morning! You can serve these with applesauce, yogurt, or salsa and avocado, or eat them as they are.

MAKES 6 PANCAKES • PREP TIME: ABOUT 30 MINUTES

1 medium zucchini, grated (about 1 cup)

1 large sweet onion, peeled and grated (about 1½ cups)

3 large Yukon gold potatoes, peeled and grated

2 eggs, beaten

¾ cup brown rice flour

¼ cup organic cornmeal

1 teaspoon Herbes de Provence or Italian seasoning

½–1 teaspoon sea salt or kosher coarse salt

½ teaspoon fresh cracked pepper, or more to taste

Up to ¼ cup coconut oil for cooking or coconut oil spray

1. Wash, peel, and grate the zucchini, onion, and potatoes. You can either do this in a food processor or with a hand grater. Drain all of the veggies on paper towels, and then squeeze out any excess water from them before transferring to a large bowl.

2. Add the beaten eggs, flour, cornmeal, herbs, salt, and pepper, and stir together well. Let this mixture sit for about 4 minutes.

3. Heat 1 tablespoon of the coconut oil over medium heat in a large skillet (or spray the skillet with coconut oil spray). When the oil is hot, drop ½ cup of mixture into the pan. Each pancake should be about ½ inch thick. Cook over medium to medium-low heat, being careful not to let the pancakes burn. Cook for 2–3 minutes on each side, or until golden brown. Continue this process until all the cakes are cooked. Drain them on paper towels prior to serving.

Note: I prefer to avoid cooking in a lot of oil, so I use a non-stick skillet and spray it lightly with coconut oil rather than frying in the oil. If you follow this method, you won't need to drain the pancakes before serving.

Italian Veggie Frittata

This dish is wonderful for a Sunday morning brunch. It is full of great flavor and will fill you up. You could easily substitute kale for the spinach if you like. If you find the veggies are sticking to the skillet during the cooking process, add a bit of vegetable stock or water to keep them from sticking.

SERVES 4 TO 6 • PREP TIME: 1 HOUR

1 tablespoon olive or coconut oil

1 medium onion, finely chopped (1 cup)

1 small shallot (optional), diced

1 cup sliced mushrooms, such as cremini or portobello

1 tablespoon chopped sun-dried tomatoes (optional)

1 medium zucchini, grated (about 1 cup)

1 cup chopped roasted red bell pepper

1 cup drained, chopped artichoke hearts

3 cups chopped spinach

1 teaspoon crushed garlic (about 2–3 cloves)

1 tablespoon dried tarragon

1½ teaspoon dried oregano

¼ teaspoon sea salt

Fresh cracked pepper to taste

6 eggs, beaten

½ cup coconut milk or other milk

¼ cup Parmesan cheese or Mock Parmesan Cheese (page 201)

1. Preheat oven to 350°F and prepare a 9 × 9-inch baking dish. Heat a large skillet (12-inch) over medium heat and add the olive oil.

2. Sauté the onions and shallots, stirring frequently, until soft, about 4 minutes. Add the mushrooms and continue cooking until they soften and begin to release their juices, about 5 minutes. Add in the sun-dried tomatoes, zucchini, roasted red bell pepper, artichoke hearts, chopped spinach, and garlic and continue to sauté, stirring often until the spinach has wilted, about 2–3 minutes. Add the herbs, salt, and pepper. Remove from heat.

3. In a medium-size bowl, beat the eggs well and add in the milk and whisk together. Add the sautéed vegetables to the egg mixture and stir to fully incorporate all of the ingredients. Pour into the 9 × 9-inch baking dish and sprinkle the top with the cheese. Bake for 40–45 minutes, or until set and lightly browned.

Tempeh Breakfast Sausage Patties

Serve these patties for breakfast alongside some breakfast muffins, eggs, or tofu scramble. Or, after cooking the patties, cut them in half and use them to fill taco shells (they taste great with lettuce, salsa, hummus, or avocado). They are quite versatile! Please note that oat flour may be unsafe for people with celiac disease (see the "Gluten-Free Oats and Oat Flour" section, page 12). If you wish to avoid oat flour or if you're unable to find GF oat flour or make your own, use teff, sorghum, or brown rice flour as a substitute.

MAKES 8 PATTIES ◆ PREP TIME: 30–40 MINUTES

1 (8-ounce) package organic GF tempeh

¼ cup GF oats

¼ cup raw sunflower seeds, ground

2 tablespoons GF oat flour

2 tablespoons tamari sauce

2 tablespoons minced onion (optional)

2 teaspoons Herbes de Provence

¼ teaspoon fresh cracked pepper

½ teaspoon sea salt

1 tablespoon coconut oil or coconut spray

1. Break the tempeh into small bite-size chunks and place them in a steamer. Steam over high heat until the tempeh is soft and cooked through, about 15 minutes.

2. When the tempeh is cooked, transfer the pieces to a large bowl. Using tongs or a fork, crumble the tempeh.

3. Add in the rest of the ingredients (except the coconut oil or spray) and blend together well, using either your hands (clean, of course) or a fork.

4. After the ingredients are mixed well, take out a handful and form it into a patty that is about 3 inches around and 1 inch thick. You should have enough ingredients to form about 8 patties, depending on their size.

5. Heat a large skillet over medium-low heat and add a small amount of coconut oil or spray, if you prefer. Cook the patties for about 4–5 minutes on each side, or until they are browned. Serve immediately. Refrigerate any leftovers.

Overnight Slow Cooker
Amaranth or Steel Cut Oats

This recipe is super easy—all you have to do is put the ingredients into the slow cooker, set it on low, and head off to bed! I don't add any sweetener to this recipe because the raisins provide enough sweetness. If you want, you can serve it with applesauce, yogurt, or berries.

SERVES 6 ◆ PREP TIME: 6–7 HOURS IN THE SLOW COOKER

8 cups water

2 cups amaranth or steel cut oats

¼ cup Medjool dates or raisins

¼ cup chopped walnuts (optional)

½–1 teaspoon cinnamon

Pinch of sea salt or kosher salt

1. Place everything in the slow cooker and stir.

2. Turn the slow cooker to low and let the oats cook for 6–7 hours overnight. Wake up and enjoy!

Granola, Granola Everywhere!

This granola recipe is one of my all-time favorites. I have made many different kinds of granola over the years, but this one is the most light and flavorful. This granola stores well for up to a month in an airtight container—but good luck keeping it around that long!

MAKES ABOUT 8 CUPS ◆ **PREP TIME: ABOUT 1 HOUR AND 30 MINUTES**

5 cups certified GF oats

1 cup chopped raw cashews

½ cup chopped raw walnuts

½ cup raisins, dates, dried
blueberries, or dried cranberries

½ cup pumpkin seeds

½ cup sesame seeds

½ cup sunflower seeds

½ cup organic maple syrup

¼ cup organic coconut oil, melted
and cooled

2 tablespoons chia seeds

2 tablespoons coconut flour (or
ground coconut flakes)

2 teaspoons cinnamon

¼ teaspoon cardamom (optional)

1. Preheat oven to 325°F.

2. Place all of the ingredients in a large mixing bowl and stir well to fully incorporate the liquid ingredients with the dry ingredients.

3. Pour half of the mixture onto a baking sheet, arranging in an even layer. Bake for about 35–40 minutes, stirring every 10–15 minutes during the baking process to ensure even cooking. Keep an eye on the granola as it's cooking so it doesn't get too dark or burned.

4. Remove the baking sheet from the oven and let the granola cool completely. Repeat the baking process with the second half of the batch.

Protein Breakfast Bars

These hearty little breakfast bars are great to eat on a plane, train, or bus, or in the car! They pack easily and can be eaten on the run, or enjoyed at home with a lovely cup of tea. The recipe is quite versatile—I added banana to this version, but that is strictly optional! If you have an allergy to nuts, use sesame seed butter and substitute the nuts for additional pumpkin seeds, sunflower seeds, or flax seeds. You can replace the almond meal for sorghum or brown rice flour too.

MAKES 10 BARS ◆ PREP TIME: ABOUT 40 MINUTES

Coconut oil spray for the baking dish

1 teaspoon chia seeds

2 tablespoons water

⅓ cup honey or brown rice syrup

1 tablespoon coconut oil

1 cup almond, peanut, or seed butter

¼ cup mashed ripe banana (optional)

2 tablespoons coconut or other milk

1 cup GF oats

½ cup almond meal (or sorghum flour)

½ cup dried cherries or cranberries

¼ cup chopped raw walnuts

¼ cup sesame seeds and pumpkin seeds

1 teaspoon vanilla extract

½ teaspoon cinnamon

¼ teaspoon sea salt

1. Preheat the oven to 325°F and lightly spray an 8 × 8-inch baking dish with coconut oil.

2. In a small bowl, whisk together the chia seeds and water and let them sit for about 5 minutes, or until gelled.

3. In a large mixing bowl, combine the honey, coconut oil, and nut butter and stir until creamy.

4. Add in the chia mixture and the rest of the ingredients and stir to fully incorporate.

5. Put the mixture into the baking dish and press it lightly to the edges with either clean hands or a wooden spoon. Bake for 25–28 minutes, or until it is golden brown and a toothpick inserted comes out clean. Cool on a wire rack. Enjoy warm from the oven, and if you have any leftovers, store them in an airtight container. They will stay fresh for several days.

Protein-Rich Seed Bars

These bars are so good you'll find yourself eating more than one! These bars are an ideal snack before exercising because they will give you a great boost of energy. They are also a perfect snack for the kids. Chia seeds will work in place of flax seeds, if you prefer. Whatever you do, keep these bars hidden or they won't last long!

MAKES 12 LARGE BARS OR 24 SMALL BARS • PREP TIME: ABOUT 1 HOUR AND 30 MINUTES

Coconut oil spray for the baking sheet

1 cup raw pumpkin seeds

1 cup raw sunflower seeds

½ cup sesame seeds

¼ cup golden flax seeds

1½ teaspoon ground cinnamon

¼ teaspoon ground ginger

⅛ teaspoon cardamom (optional)

1 teaspoon vanilla extract

⅓ cup brown rice syrup

1. Preheat oven to 300°F. Lightly spray a rimmed baking sheet with coconut oil.

2. Place all of the seeds and spices into a large bowl, add the vanilla extract, and stir with a wooden spoon. Drizzle the brown rice syrup over the mixture and stir to fully blend together. This mixture is sticky and may be difficult to mix, but do your best to fully blend everything together.

3. Pour the mixture onto your prepared baking sheet. With clean and damp hands, press the mixture out into a large rectangle (about 8 x 12 inches). Bake for 40–45 minutes. Halfway through the baking time, use a large wooden spoon to flatten the mixture to the baking sheet. This will help it hold together when cooled.

4. Remove the baking sheet from the oven and let it cool for about 30 minutes before cutting with a sharp knife into bars. These bars can be stored in a ziplock plastic bag or an airtight container. They will go quickly, but if you happen to have any leftovers, they store well for up to a week.

Breads, Muffins, and Scones

Hearty Sandwich Bread

This bread doesn't rise up as high as traditional wheat bread, but it is a perfect bread for toast or sandwiches because it doesn't fall apart. I like making open-faced sandwiches with grilled veggies, and I love using this bread for them—this hearty bread holds up well and has a great flavor.

MAKES ONE 9-INCH LOAF   ◆   PREP TIME: 1 HOUR AND 15 MINUTES

Coconut oil spray for the loaf pan

1 tablespoon active dry yeast

¼ cup warm water

1 teaspoon coconut palm sugar (optional)

1 cup brown rice flour

¼ cup coconut flour

½ cup almond meal (store-bought, or see recipe on page 195)

¾ cup raw, unsalted sunflower seeds

¼ cup golden flax seeds

¾ teaspoon sea salt

¾ cup arrowroot powder

1 tablespoon guar gum

2 eggs

2 egg whites, separated

1 tablespoon apple cider vinegar

½ cup coconut, soy, or hemp milk

¼ cup olive oil

¼ cup molasses

1. Prepare a 9-inch bread loaf pan by lightly spraying it with coconut oil and set it aside.

2. Put the yeast in a large bowl and add the warm water. If using the sugar to help activate the yeast, sprinkle it on top and let it sit until it bubbles, up to 10 minutes.

3. While the yeast is activating, in a separate bowl mix together the dry ingredients: flours, almond meal, seeds, salt, arrowroot powder, and guar gum.

4. In a different small bowl, whisk the eggs, egg whites, vinegar, milk, oil, and molasses together well. Add this egg mixture to the large bowl with the yeast and stir.

5. Add the dry ingredients to the wet mixture and beat together with an electric mixer on low speed for 1–2 minutes. Scrape down the sides of the bowl and then blend at a medium-high speed for 2–3 minutes.

6. Put all of the bread mixture into the prepared loaf pan. Cover the pan with a lightweight tea towel or aluminum foil and set it aside in a warm spot to allow it to rise for about 40 minutes. While the bread is rising, preheat the oven to 350°F. (See note below for a tip on how to speed up the rising process.)

7. After the loaf has risen to about an inch below the top of the pan, put it into the oven and bake it for 45–50 minutes. The bread will be lightly browned and should sound hollow when tapped lightly. Take the bread out of the oven and let it rest in the loaf pan for 10 minutes. Then remove the bread from the loaf pan and cool it on a wire rack.

continues

continued

Notes: There is a way you can speed up the rising process if you wish. Preheat the oven to 200°F, then turn it off. Open the oven door and make sure the oven is not too hot, just warm. Place the uncovered loaf pan in the oven. The dough will rise in about 30 minutes. If you use this method, wait until the dough is fully risen before changing the temperature to 350°F for baking.

To make your own coconut flour, place a cup of organic shredded coconut in a food processor and pulse until the coconut is the consistency of flour. Store the coconut flour in an airtight container in the refrigerator and use it in place of store-bought coconut flour, if desired.

Buckwheat Bread

This hearty bread has a great flavor due to the combination of the buckwheat and almond flours. It is not too heavy, but it really fills you up. Store it in an airtight container at room temperature, and it will stay fresh for a few days. For best results, toast this bread after it is two days old.

MAKES ONE 8-INCH LOAF ◆ **PREP TIME: 65–70 MINUTES**

Coconut oil spray for the loaf pan

1½ tablespoons active dry yeast

½ cup plus 1¼ cups warm water

1 teaspoon (optional) plus
　2 teaspoons coconut palm sugar

2 eggs

1 teaspoon sea salt

1 teaspoon baking powder

1 tablespoons chia seeds or flax
　seeds

2 tablespoons almond meal

1 cup sorghum flour

2 cups buckwheat flour

1. Prepare an 8-inch loaf pan by lightly spraying it with coconut oil and set it aside.

2. Place the yeast in a large bowl and add ½ cup warm water. If you wish to use the sugar to help activate the yeast, sprinkle 1 teaspoon of the sugar on top and let it sit for up to 10 minutes.

3. While the yeast is activating, beat the eggs and the remaining 1¼ cups of warm water in a small mixing bowl. Add the egg mixture to the yeast and stir to mix together.

4. In a large bowl, combine all of the dry ingredients, including the remaining 2 teaspoons coconut sugar, salt, baking powder, seeds, almond meal, sorghum flour, and buckwheat flour. Whisk together to combine.

5. Add the dry ingredients to the yeast mixture and use a wooden spoon to stir well, until the ingredients combine into a dough.

6. Place the dough in the prepared loaf pan and cover it with a lightweight tea towel or aluminum foil. Set it in a warm place to rise. The dough will rise to about an inch from the top of the loaf pan in about 30–40 minutes.

7. While the dough rises, preheat oven to 350°F. When the dough is ready, bake it for about 30 minutes. Tap lightly on the top of the loaf to be sure it is done—the loaf should sound hollow when tapped. Cool it on a wire rack.

Butternut Squash or Zucchini Bread

This recipe is amazing! It can be made with butternut squash or zucchini, and the dough can be baked into bread, muffins, or cake. I recently used this recipe for a cake (in a 9 × 9-inch pan) and it was delicious—no frosting necessary! If you use eggs in this recipe, the bread will be very light; if you wish to make this recipe vegan, use 2 teaspoons of chia seeds mixed with 4 teaspoons of water as a substitute. The vegan bread will be much denser but just as delicious!

MAKES ONE 8-INCH LOAF ◆ **PREP TIME: IF USING ZUCCHINI, THIS RECIPE WILL TAKE 45–55 MINUTES TO PREPARE. IF USING BUTTERNUT SQUASH, ADD AN ADDITIONAL 30–40 MINUTES FOR ROASTING THE SQUASH.**

Coconut oil spray for the loaf pan

2 medium zucchinis or 1 medium butternut squash (about 1½ cups of zucchini or squash)

1 cup almond meal or flour (page 195)

½ cup sorghum flour

1 teaspoon baking soda

2 teaspoons baking powder

1 teaspoon guar gum (optional)

¼ teaspoon sea salt

1 heaping teaspoon cinnamon

½ teaspoon nutmeg (freshly ground if possible)

½ cup organic coconut palm sugar

¼ cup coconut oil

2 eggs (or 2 teaspoons chia seeds whisked with 4 tablespoons water; allow 5–6 minutes to gel)

½ cup coconut milk (not concentrate)

1 tablespoon organic maple syrup

2 teaspoons vanilla extract

½ cup walnuts, chopped

1. Preheat the oven to 350°F. Prepare an 8 × 4½-inch loaf pan by lightly spraying it with coconut oil.

2. If you're using the fresh zucchini, grate it and skip directly to step 3. If you're using the butternut squash, you'll need to roast it first. Cut the top and bottom off of the butternut squash and slice it directly down the center. Scoop out the seeds and place the squash, face down, on a baking sheet that has been lightly sprayed with coconut oil or olive oil. Use a fork to poke the skin of the squash all over and then bake it in the oven at 375°F until soft, between 30–40 minutes, depending on the size of the squash. To make sure it's done, stick a knife through the squash; the knife should slide through easily if the squash is fully cooked. Remove the squash from the oven and set it aside to cool. When the squash is cool enough to touch, peel off the skin and place the squash in a bowl. Use a fork to mash the squash. Set aside.

3. In a medium-size bowl, combine the flours, baking soda, baking powder, guar gum (optional), salt, cinnamon, and nutmeg together and whisk to blend well.

4. In a large mixing bowl, use an electric mixer on medium speed to blend together the sugar and coconut oil, about 1 minute. Add the eggs (or chia seed mixture), milk, maple syrup, and vanilla extract and mix on medium speed to blend ingredients, about 2 minutes.

5. Add the dry ingredients to the wet mixture and stir with the mixer to combine well.

6. Add in the squash (or zucchini) and nuts and stir with a wooden spoon to fully incorporate.

7. Pour the dough into the prepared loaf pan and bake for approximately 43–45 minutes. To make sure the bread is cooked all the way through, poke the loaf with a toothpick or sharp knife—it should come out clean. Remove the bread from the oven and place it on a cooling rack. Cool it in the pan for 10–15 minutes, then take a knife and carefully go around the sides of the bread to ease it out of the pan. Cool it on a wire rack. This bread will store well in an airtight container and will stay fresh if stored properly for several days.

Note: If you use zucchini in this recipe, you will use raw, grated zucchini. However, if you use butternut squash, you will need to roast it first and then mash the cooked squash prior to adding to the recipe.

Pumpkin and Banana Bread

This bread is very moist and delicious. It is made with almond meal, which adds protein and complex carbohydrates. The coconut cream can be found in health-food stores or at Trader Joe's, or you can make your own with a fresh coconut by blending the coconut meat with water. If you are allergic to nuts, substitute sorghum flour for the almond meal. If you are a vegan and do not want to use eggs, replace the egg with 1 teaspoon chia seeds whisked with 2 tablespoons water; let the chia mixture sit for 5–6 minutes to gel before adding it to the liquid ingredients.

MAKES ONE 9-INCH LOAF • PREP TIME: 1 HOUR

Coconut oil spray for the loaf pan

½ cup vegan margarine

½ cup organic coconut palm sugar

¼ cup mashed ripe banana

¼ cup coconut cream

1 teaspoon vanilla extract

1 egg (or chia seeds replacement, see headnote)

1 cup organic pumpkin purée

1 cup almond meal

1 cup brown rice flour

¼ teaspoon sea salt

1½ teaspoons cinnamon

2 teaspoons baking powder

1 teaspoon baking soda

1. Preheat the oven to 350°F and lightly spray a 6 × 9-inch loaf pan with coconut oil.

2. In a large mixer, combine the margarine and sugar and beat until well blended and light and fluffy. Add the banana, coconut cream, vanilla extract, and egg and continue to beat together for about 1–2 minutes. Add the pumpkin and beat on high for 1 minute.

3. In a small bowl, combine the almond meal, brown rice flour, salt, cinnamon, baking powder, and baking soda and stir to blend well. Add the dry ingredients to the wet ingredients all at once and mix on medium speed to fully incorporate.

4. Pour the dough into the prepared loaf pan. Bake for about 45–50 minutes, or until a sharp knife or toothpick comes out clean. Cool on a wire rack for about 30 minutes, then remove from the pan. This bread stores well in an airtight container for several days, if it's not eaten by then!

Coconut and Pumpkin Bread

Pumpkin is good for us because it's chock-full of nutrients, including vitamins A, C, K, and E, and it's also a good source of minerals, such as potassium, iron, and magnesium. And it's also a complex carbohydrate. Another wonderful thing about pumpkins is that even though they grow in the fall, they don't have to just be a fall vegetable. Pumpkins store well for up to six months in a cool, dry place. In my grandmother's day, pumpkins would have been stored in a cellar, but these days, you can keep your pumpkins in the garage, basement, or other cool, dry location. If you use organic canned pumpkin, it's available year-round!

MAKES ONE 9-INCH LOAF • PREP TIME: 1 HOUR; ADD 45 MINUTES IF USING FRESH PUMPKIN

Coconut oil spray for the loaf pan

1 cup organic pumpkin purée (or 1 small pumpkin, if using fresh) or other squash purée

½ cup organic coconut palm sugar

½ cup vegan margarine (or butter)

¼ cup mashed ripe banana

1 teaspoon vanilla extract

1 egg (or 1 teaspoon chia seeds whisked with 2 tablespoons water; allow 5–6 minutes to gel)

¼ cup coconut cream

1 cup brown rice flour

1 cup almond meal

2 teaspoons baking powder

1 teaspoon baking soda

1½ teaspoons ground cinnamon

¼ teaspoon sea salt

1. Preheat the oven to 350°F and lightly spray a 9 × 5-inch loaf pan with coconut oil.

2. If you're using organic canned pumpkin, skip to step 3. If you're using fresh pumpkin, choose a small one so it's sweet and won't take too long to bake. Cut the top off and then slice the pumpkin in half lengthwise. Scoop out the seeds and discard them (or keep them for another purpose). Quarter the pumpkin and place it on a baking sheet, face up. Bake in a 350°F oven for about 40–45 minutes, or until fork tender. When the pumpkin is cool, scoop it out of the skin and purée it in a food processor until smooth.

3. In a large mixing bowl, cream together the sugar and margarine with a hand mixer or an electric mixer until light and fluffy. Add in the mashed banana, vanilla extract, and egg (or egg substitute) and beat well to combine. Add the pumpkin purée and coconut cream and blend well.

4. In a small bowl, combine the flour and almond meal, baking powder, baking soda, cinnamon, and salt. Add the dry ingredients to the wet ingredients and stir on medium speed to blend together, about 1 minute.

5. Pour the dough into the loaf pan and bake for 45–50 minutes, or until a toothpick or sharp knife comes out clean. Cool the bread on a wire rack completely before slicing. Store in an airtight container. Will stay fresh for several days.

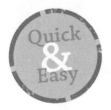

Protein-Packed
Carrot Muffins

I like muffins that pack a protein punch! These muffins, with their lentil base and other healthy ingredients, have tons of protein. If you have an allergy to nuts, please substitute the almond meal with additional sorghum flour or garbanzo bean flour. Send these muffins to school with the kids for an afternoon energy boost!

MAKES 12 MUFFINS • PREP TIME: 30 MINUTES

¾ cup red lentils, rinsed

1½ cups water

½ cup sorghum flour

½ cup garbanzo bean flour

¾ cup almond meal

1 tablespoon chia seeds

1½ teaspoons baking powder

1 teaspoon baking soda

2 teaspoons ground cinnamon

1 teaspoon guar gum

¼ teaspoon sea salt

¼ cup coconut oil

⅓ cup honey or maple syrup

¼ cup organic coconut palm sugar

⅔ cup unsweetened applesauce

1 cup grated carrot

1. After rinsing the lentils, place them in a saucepan and cover them with the water. Bring the water to a boil over high heat, then reduce the heat and simmer over medium-low heat for about 8–10 minutes, or until lentils are cooked through. Set them aside to cool. Drain any excess liquid from the lentils and purée them in a food processor or blender until smooth.

2. Preheat the oven to 350°F. Lightly spray a muffin tin with coconut oil or line the muffin tin with paper muffin cups.

3. In a large mixing bowl, whisk together the flours, almond meal, chia seeds, baking powder, baking soda, cinnamon, guar gum, and salt.

4. In a separate mixing bowl, combine the oil, honey (or maple syrup), and sugar and beat well. Add in the applesauce and carrots and blend together. Add the wet mixture to the dry ingredients and stir until well combined.

5. Fill the prepared muffin cups about halfway with batter. Bake for 18–20 minutes, or until a toothpick or sharp knife inserted in the center of a muffin comes out clean. Cool the muffins on a wire rack, then remove them from the pan. Store any leftover muffins in an airtight container or freeze them for later use. These will freeze well for up to a month.

Lemon and Berry Muffins

Not only are these muffins delicious, but they are also nutritious! You will feel good about serving them to your family because they are made with garbanzo flour, which is full of protein. The recipe calls for a blend of sorghum and garbanzo flours, but you can use all garbanzo flour, if preferred! I like to use raspberries in these muffins, but blueberries would pair nicely with the lemon flavor too!

MAKES 12 MUFFINS • PREP TIME: 30–40 MINUTES

½ cup sorghum flour (can substitute all bean flour if preferred)

¾ cup garbanzo bean flour

2 teaspoons baking powder

½ teaspoon baking soda

1 teaspoon guar gum

¼ teaspoon sea salt

1 teaspoon chia seeds

2 tablespoons water

¼ cup coconut oil

½ cup maple syrup (or brown rice syrup) or coconut palm sugar

½ cup coconut, soy, or hemp milk

2 tablespoons lemon juice, freshly squeezed if possible

1 cup fresh or frozen raspberries

1. Preheat the oven to 375°F. Lightly spray the cups of a muffin tin with coconut oil spray or line the muffin tin with paper muffin cups.

2. In a large bowl, combine the sorghum flour, garbanzo bean flour, baking powder, baking soda, guar gum, and salt. Blend together well.

3. In a different large mixing bowl, combine the chia seeds with the water and whisk together well. Let this mixture sit for about 5–6 minutes to gel.

4. Add the oil, maple syrup, milk, and lemon juice to the chia mixture and beat well.

5. Add the wet ingredients to the dry ingredients and stir together until fully incorporated. Fold in the raspberries.

6. Fill the prepared muffin cups about halfway with batter. Bake for 25–30 minutes, or until a toothpick or sharp knife inserted in the center of a muffin comes out clean. Cool the muffins on a wire rack, then remove them from the pan. Store muffins in an airtight container. The muffins will stay fresh for 2–3 days.

Note: This recipe is vegan. If you wish to add eggs to the recipe, omit the chia seeds and water and replace them with one beaten egg.

Oat and Walnut Scones

These scones are delicious topped with a drizzle of honey or your favorite jam. To vary the flavor of this recipe, you can reduce the milk by ¼ cup and add orange juice and a pinch of cardamom if you like. Please note that this recipe calls for oat flour, which may be unsafe for people with celiac disease. If you are buying oat flour, please be sure that it is gluten-free! Another option is to make your own oat flour by putting GF oats into a food processor and pulsing until the mixture is fine like flour. You can use the flour immediately, or store it in an airtight container in your refrigerator for future use.

MAKES 8 SCONES • PREP TIME: 45 MINUTES OR LESS

1 teaspoon chia seeds

2 tablespoons water

1 cup GF oat flour

¾ cup brown rice flour or sorghum flour

½ cup arrowroot powder

¼ cup GF oats

1 teaspoon guar gum (optional)

1 tablespoon baking powder

¼ teaspoon sea salt

1 tablespoon organic coconut palm sugar

1½ teaspoons cinnamon

¼ cup raw walnuts, chopped

5 tablespoons butter, thinly sliced

2 egg whites plus 1 egg yolk

½ cup coconut, hemp, or other milk

1. Preheat the oven to 400°F. Have an ungreased baking sheet ready.

2. While the oven is heating up, combine the chia seeds and water in a small bowl and whisk together well. Set aside for about 5–6 minutes to allow the mixture to gel.

3. In a large bowl, whisk together all of the dry ingredients, including the flours, arrowroot powder, oats, guar gum, baking powder, salt, sugar, cinnamon, and nuts. Cut in the butter with a pastry blender, a fork, or your clean fingers, until the butter is incorporated.

4. In a separate bowl, use an electric mixer to beat the egg whites until they are light and fluffy.

5. Add the egg yolk and milk to the chia seed mixture and whisk together. Then add this mixture to the dry ingredients and stir to blend. Gently fold in egg whites. Do not over-mix the dough or the scones will be tough when baked. Only mix together gently until the ingredients are fully incorporated.

6. Line a work surface with parchment paper or brown rice flour. Turn the dough out and form a large circle, patting it with your hands until it is about an inch or so thick. Use a sharp knife to cut the circle into eight equal pieces, like you would a pie. Do so by cutting the circle in half lengthwise, then in half again, continuing until you have eight equal pieces. Do not pull the pieces apart; they will be baked together in the circle and separated after they are taken out of the oven.

7. Carefully slide the parchment paper with the scones onto the baking sheet and put them in the oven. Reduce the heat to 375°F and bake for 25–30 minutes, or until the scones are lightly browned and cooked all the way through. The scones should be firm to touch. Remove the baking sheet from the oven. Cut the scones apart and place them on a wire rack to cool. They can be stored in an airtight container and will stay fresh for a day or two at the most.

Teff and Berry Scones

For this scone recipe, I used three different flours: mainly teff flour and sorghum flour, with a small amount of coconut flour for flavor. If you don't have coconut flour on hand, don't sweat it! Put a small amount of organic flaked coconut into a food processor and pulse it until it is fine like flour. Or, don't use coconut, and increase the sorghum flour to 2 cups instead. If you are a vegan and do not want to use eggs, simply replace the egg with 1 teaspoon chia seeds whisked together with 2 tablespoons water; allow the mixture to sit for 5–6 minutes to gel before adding to the liquid ingredients.

MAKES ABOUT 16 SCONES • PREP TIME: 30–35 MINUTES

2 cups teff flour

1½ cups sorghum flour

½ cup coconut flour

1 cup arrowroot powder

2 teaspoons guar gum

1 heaping teaspoon cinnamon

1 teaspoon baking powder

1 teaspoon baking soda

½ teaspoon sea salt

½ cup coconut oil, melted

½ cup maple syrup

1 egg

1½ teaspoons vanilla extract

¼ cup unsweetened applesauce

1¼–1½ cups coconut milk (or hemp or other non-dairy milk)

2 cups fresh or frozen strawberries, raspberries, or blueberries

1. Preheat oven to 350°F. Cover a large cookie sheet with parchment paper.

2. In a large bowl, stir together the dry ingredients until well blended.

3. In a separate bowl, combine the coconut oil (allow your melted oil to cool before you use it), maple syrup, egg, vanilla extract, applesauce, and milk and whisk together well.

4. Add the wet ingredients to the dry ingredients and stir well. Fold in the berries gently and stir until incorporated; do not over-mix. The dough will be somewhat dry but should hold its shape when scooped.

5. Using your clean hands, form the dough into 2½-inch balls. You can shape them into either round balls or triangles. You should have enough dough for about 16 scones. Place the scones on the prepared cookie sheet and bake for 25 minutes, or until the edges are browned slightly. Remove from the pan and cool on a wire rack. Store the scones in an airtight container, and they will stay fresh for a day or two. I often freeze them in a ziplock plastic bag and then serve them at a later date with tea. They freeze well and can be frozen for several weeks.

Soups
and Salads

Healing Miso Soup

Miso contains all of the essential amino acids and is a complete protein. It contains beneficial prebiotics, helps in digestion, and is a great source of B-vitamins and antioxidants. It also helps to strengthen the immune system. If feel you run down or a bit under the weather, make this soup! It is so warm and nurturing. It's the perfect soup to serve on a cold winter's night alongside a fresh green salad. If you want to make the soup more substantial, add a cup of cooked quinoa, GF soba noodles, or brown rice.

SERVES 2 TO 3   ♦   PREP TIME: 30–40 MINUTES

1 tablespoon organic olive oil

1 medium sweet onion, finely chopped (about 1 cup)

1 cup stemmed, chopped cremini mushrooms

1 tablespoon finely chopped fresh garlic

1 tablespoon grated fresh ginger

5–6 cups water

4 tablespoons organic, GF red miso paste

Salt and fresh cracked pepper to taste

Pinch of red pepper flakes or cayenne pepper (optional)

1. Heat a large skillet over medium-high heat and add the olive oil.

2. Sauté the onion until soft, about 4–5 minutes. Add in the mushrooms, garlic, and ginger and continue to cook until the ginger and garlic is soft, about 5 minutes or longer, if needed.

3. While the veggies cook, pour the water into a large stock pot and add the miso paste. Whisk vigorously until the miso is dissolved. When the veggies are done, add them to the miso broth and bring the soup to a low boil. Turn down the heat to low and simmer for 15–20 minutes.

4. Pour the soup from the stock pot into a blender and blend it until the vegetables are puréed. Return the soup to the stock pot and heat through on low. Season with fresh cracked pepper and salt. If you want your soup to have more of a kick, add red pepper flakes or cayenne pepper and stir. Serve immediately.

Mock French Onion Soup with Mushrooms

I love onion soup, so I wanted to develop a tasty onion base without using beef broth. This soup is great without the bread or cheese found on traditional French onion soup, but if you do want to dress your soup up in the traditional way without the gluten, then I recommend broiling a piece of GF bread on both sides, cutting it into cubes, and topping your bowl of soup with the bread cubes. Then sprinkle mozzarella or a dairy-free cheese substitute on top and broil the whole bowl for a few minutes, until the cheese is bubbly and browned.

SERVES 4 • PREP TIME: 60–75 MINUTES

3 tablespoons butter or vegan margarine

1 tablespoon olive oil

5 cups finely chopped sweet onions

2 cups sliced cremini mushrooms

1 tablespoon garlic

½ cup red wine (Cabernet, or vegetable stock if you prefer)

4 cups mushroom stock (page 192) or vegetable stock (page 193)

1½ cups water

1 tablespoon red miso paste

2 tablespoons chopped fresh parsley

Pinch of thyme

½ teaspoon fresh cracked pepper

Sea salt to taste

1. Heat the butter and olive oil in a large Dutch oven or soup pot over medium heat.

2. Add the onions and cook slowly for 20 minutes, stirring frequently. You want to slowly caramelize the onions, so if they are beginning to brown too quickly, reduce the heat or add 1–2 tablespoons mushroom or vegetable stock. (If you cook the onions on medium or medium-low heat, you shouldn't have to add the stock.)

3. Add the mushrooms and continue cooking for another 5 minutes. Add the garlic and cook for 5 more minutes, stirring frequently. Your onions should now be golden brown and the mushrooms should be soft.

4. Add the wine, mushroom stock, water, miso, parsley, and thyme and simmer for 20–30 minutes. Season with fresh cracked pepper and salt. Serve immediately.

Thai Vegetable and Quinoa Soup

The combination of coconut milk and red curry paste in this soup gives it a soothing taste. You can spice up the soup by adding 1–2 teaspoons of chopped jalapeño. The fresh ginger and garlic in this soup act to boost your immune system, so eat it in the wintertime for the added bonus of warding off germs!

SERVES 6 • PREP TIME: 30–45 MINUTES

1 tablespoon coconut oil

1 cup finely chopped onion

1 cup diced fresh green beans

½ cup chopped carrots

1 cup chopped kale

1½ cups chopped baby bok choy

¾ cup sliced cremini mushrooms

2 tablespoons thinly sliced fresh ginger

1 tablespoon minced garlic

4 cups vegetable stock (page 193)

2 cups water

1 tablespoon plus 2 teaspoons red curry paste

2 tablespoons tamari sauce

⅓ cup chopped fresh cilantro

½ teaspoon cumin

¼ teaspoon turmeric

¼ teaspoon ground coriander

Large pinch of red pepper flakes

1–2 teaspoons finely chopped jalapeño pepper (optional)

¾ cup canned organic coconut milk

1 tablespoon fresh lime juice

1 cup cooked quinoa (cook according to package directions)

Sea salt and fresh cracked pepper to taste

1. Heat a large stock pot or Dutch oven on medium and add the coconut oil.

2. When the oil is hot, add the onion and sauté until soft, about 4 minutes. Add in the green beans and carrots and continue to sauté for another 4–5 minutes, or until they are beginning to soften but are not completely cooked through. Add in the kale and baby bok choy and continue to sauté for another 2–3 minutes. Add the mushrooms, ginger, and garlic and sauté for 2 minutes.

3. Add the vegetable stock, water, red curry paste, tamari, and seasonings to the stock pot or Dutch oven. Reduce the heat to medium-low and simmer for 20 minutes.

4. Add in the coconut milk, lime juice, and cooked quinoa. Simmer until the soup is heated through. Season with salt and fresh cracked pepper to taste. Serve immediately.

Curried Lentil and Spinach Soup

Lentils are low in calories and provide soluble fiber, which is known to reduce blood cholesterol. Lentils are also a great source of foliate and magnesium, and 26 percent of the calories in lentils are attributed to protein. They are easy to cook and have a unique nutty taste. If you want to make the soup creamier, consider adding the optional coconut cream to the recipe.

SERVES 6 TO 8 • PREP TIME: ABOUT 1 HOUR

2 tablespoons coconut oil

1 cup chopped onion

1 large carrot, chopped

2 celery stalks, chopped

2 cups chopped fresh spinach

1 cup lentils, cleaned and rinsed (red or green)

2 cups vegetable stock (page 193)

1 (6-ounce) can organic tomato paste

2 cups water

½ teaspoon sea salt, or more to taste

1 tablespoon curry powder

¼ teaspoon ground coriander

¼ teaspoon cumin

2 tablespoons coconut cream (optional)

¼ cup green onions (garnish, optional)

1. In a large Dutch oven or stock pot, heat the oil over medium-high heat.

2. Add the onion, carrot, and celery and sauté until soft, about 5 minutes. Add in the spinach and continue to sauté for another minute.

3. Add the lentils, vegetable stock, tomato paste, water, and seasonings and stir well. Bring the mixture to a boil and then reduce the heat to medium-low and cover. Cook the mixture for about 15–20 minutes, or until the lentils are tender.

4. If desired, add the coconut cream and stir to blend it in. Garnish with the green onions, if you wish. Serve immediately.

Quick Savoy Cabbage Soup
with Rice or Quinoa

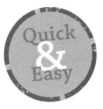

This tasty soup is hearty and filling, and surprisingly simple to make. You can put this soup together quickly by using pre-cooked rice or quinoa—this recipe is a great choice when you want to use up your leftover grains. Please note that if you are starting the recipe with uncooked rice or quinoa, you'll need to adjust your cooking time. If you are adding uncooked brown rice to the soup, add 35 minutes to your simmer time; for uncooked quinoa, add an extra 10 minutes.

SERVES 4 • PREP TIME: ABOUT 30 MINUTES

1 tablespoon coconut oil

1 cup finely chopped onion

¾ cup chopped carrot

5 cups chopped savoy cabbage

2 cloves garlic, minced

2 cups water

4 cups vegetable stock (page 193)

1 tablespoon tamari

1 cup cooked brown or red rice or quinoa

Dash of red pepper flakes

Sea salt and fresh cracked pepper to taste

1. Heat a stock pot or Dutch oven over medium heat and add the oil.

2. When the oil is hot, add the onion and carrots and sauté for 4 minutes, or until the onion is soft. Add the cabbage and garlic and continue to sauté for another 2–3 minutes, or until the cabbage is slightly wilted.

3. Add the water, vegetable stock, and tamari and simmer on medium-low heat for 10 minutes, or until the cabbage is cooked. Add the cooked rice or quinoa, red pepper flakes, salt, and pepper and simmer until the soup is heated through, about 3–4 minutes. If you're starting with uncooked grains, please see the instructions in the headnote about adjusting the simmer time.

Mushroom and Chard Soup

This filling and nutritious soup provides a simple meal that is easy to prepare. The soup is made with a few straightforward ingredients, and it doesn't have any big, overpowering flavors. If you would like to dress it up a bit, use Parmesan cheese or Mock Parmesan Cheese (recipe on page 201) to sprinkle on top of each bowl before serving.

SERVES 4 • PREP TIME: 30–45 MINUTES

1 tablespoon olive oil

1 cup chopped onion

4 cups chopped Swiss chard

1 pound cremini mushrooms, cleaned, stemmed, and cut in half

2 cups cooked white beans

2 tablespoons Bragg's Liquid Amino Acids

2 cups mushroom stock (page 192)

2 cups water

Red pepper flakes

Pinch of dried rosemary

Sea salt and fresh cracked pepper to taste

1. In a Dutch oven or stock pot, heat the olive oil over medium-high heat.

2. When the oil is hot, add the onion and sauté it for 3–4 minutes, or until soft. Add the chard and continue to sauté for another 3–4 minutes, until the chard is wilted. Add the mushrooms and continue to sauté until they are soft, about 4–5 minutes.

3. Add the beans, Bragg's Amino Acids, mushroom stock, water, red pepper flakes, and rosemary and stir together. Turn the heat down to medium-low and let the soup simmer for 20–30 minutes. Season with salt and pepper to taste. Serve immediately.

Note: This recipe calls for Bragg's Amino Acids. If you do not wish to use Bragg's Amino Acids in the recipe, feel free to use GF tamari sauce as a substitute.

Vegetable and Tempeh Pho

Pho (pronounced fuh) is a Vietnamese noodle soup traditionally made with meat. I have developed a vegetarian version that includes tempeh or tofu; if you don't eat soy, just leave it out. Pho is easy to make and quite filling. If you like a lot of spice, add some hot sauce to this soup and really fire up your immune system!

SERVES 4 TO 6 • PREP TIME: 45–60 MINUTES

1 tablespoon coconut oil or olive oil

1 cup chopped onion

1 cup crumbled GF tempeh or tofu

1 cup chopped Swiss chard

½ cup sliced carrots

2 cups chopped bok choy

2 cups sliced cremini mushrooms

4 cloves garlic, minced (about 1 tablespoon)

1 tablespoon grated fresh ginger

1 medium jalapeño, de-seeded and chopped (about 1–2 tablespoons)

4 cups vegetable stock or a combination of mushroom/vegetable stock (see pages 192 and 193)

2 cups water

½ cup chopped fresh basil

1–2 tablespoons chopped fresh cilantro

¼ cup lime juice

1 tablespoon red miso paste

1 tablespoon rice wine vinegar

3 tablespoons GF tamari

Sea salt to taste

1 teaspoon fresh cracked pepper

16 ounces kelp noodles (about 2 cups) or 8 ounces flat rice noodles

Lime slices, for garnish

¼–½ cup whole basil leaves, for garnish

4 green scallions, for garnish

1 cup bean sprouts, for garnish

1. Heat a Dutch oven or a large stock pot over medium heat and add the oil.

2. When the oil is hot, add the onion and sauté it for 4 minutes, or until it is soft, stirring occasionally. Add the tempeh or tofu, chard, carrots, and bok choy, and continue to sauté for another 2–3 minutes. Add the mushrooms, garlic, ginger, and jalapeño pepper and sauté for an additional 3–4 minutes.

3. Add the vegetable stock, water, herbs, lime juice, miso, vinegar, tamari, salt, and pepper, then reduce heat to medium-low and simmer for 30 minutes.

4. While the soup simmers, prepare the noodles. Kelp noodles don't need to be cooked, but rinse them well. If you are using rice noodles, cook them according to the directions on the package, then drain and rinse them.

5. When you're ready to serve the soup, put a helping of noodles into a bowl and pour the soup over the top. Serve with a plate of lime slices, green scallions, basil leaves, and bean sprouts.

Slow Cooker Curry Vegetable Stew

This is such an easy dinner to make because your slow cooker does most of the work! All you need to do is wash and chop the ingredients and put them into the slow cooker, and voilá! I love serving this over polenta, quinoa, or rice, but it's also good by itself or garnished with fresh mint. For the red curry paste, I like to use the brand Thai Kitchen, which can be found in the condiment section of the supermarket. If you can't find it at the grocery store, try a local Asian market or a health-food store such as Whole Foods or Mother's Market. They will have it!

SERVES 6 TO 8 ◆ PREP TIME: ABOUT 10–15 MINUTES TO PREPARE AND 3 HOURS TO COOK

3 cups cooked chickpeas, drained

1 large cauliflower head, chopped into bite-size chunks (about 4 cups)

2 cups chopped (1-inch pieces) squash (I use a combination of summer squash and zucchini)

1 cup baby carrots

1 teaspoon minced garlic

1 cup chopped red or yellow onion

1 cup diced Yukon gold potatoes

½ cup water

2 cups tomato sauce

¼ cup red wine vinegar

2 tablespoons thinly sliced fresh ginger

2 teaspoons cumin

1 teaspoon red curry paste

2 tablespoons curry powder

1 teaspoon cinnamon

Salt and fresh cracked pepper to taste

Fresh mint or cilantro, for garnish

1. Put all of the ingredients into a slow cooker (4–5 quarts) and cook on high heat for 3 hours. Stir the stew halfway through the cooking time, if you wish, or leave it alone until it is done cooking. Serve and top with mint or cilantro, if desired.

Mung Bean Stew

According to the Chinese herbal pharmacist and author Li Shizhen, mung beans are not only a great source of nutrients, they can also be used to clear toxins from the body. One cup of mung beans contains 31 calories, zero grams of fat, 2 grams of fiber, 3 grams of protein, and 4 grams of sugar. Additionally, they are high in vitamin K, vitamin C, iron, and calcium. Mung beans can also be sprouted, and the sprouts are great on panini sandwiches, salads, stir-fries, soups, and casseroles.

SERVES 4 • PREP TIME: 1 HOUR, PLUS SOAKING TIME

2 cups dry mung beans

1 tablespoon coconut oil

1 cup finely chopped onion

1 cup finely chopped carrots

3–4 cloves garlic, minced

1 cup finely chopped celery

2 cups chopped kale

4 cups vegetable stock (page 193)

4 cups water

¼ cup red wine (optional)

2 bay leaves

1 teaspoon minced fresh ginger

1 teaspoon cumin

½ teaspoon coriander

½ teaspoon dried oregano

Sea salt and fresh cracked pepper to taste

1. Soak mung beans for at least 8 hours, or overnight. Drain the beans and rinse them well. Set them aside.

2. In a large stock pot or Dutch oven, heat the oil over medium heat.

3. When the oil is hot, add the onion and sauté it until it is soft, about 4 minutes. Add the carrots, garlic, celery, and kale and continue to sauté for 4–5 minutes, or until the kale is wilted.

4. Add the vegetable stock, water, wine, seasonings (except for the salt and pepper), and mung beans and bring it to a boil. Once the soup boils, reduce the heat to a low simmer and cook for about 45 minutes, or until the beans are tender.

5. Transfer half of the soup mixture into a blender and purée it for about a minute, until the soup is thick. Return it to the stock pot or Dutch oven and cook it until it's heated through. Season the soup with salt and fresh cracked pepper to taste and serve.

Slow Cooker Lentil Vegetable Soup

All this recipe requires is some washing and chopping, then you put all of the ingredients into the slow cooker and GO! I've suggested a tasty combination of vegetables, but feel free to substitute these with any other vegetables you have on hand. Soups are a great way to use up veggies so they don't go to waste—and you end up with a nutritious, ready-to-serve meal!

SERVES 6 • PREP TIME: 15 MINUTES TO PREP AND 6 HOURS IN THE SLOW COOKER

1 cup chopped onion

4 cups chopped cauliflower

3 cups chopped savoy cabbage

1 cup chopped carrots

2 cups chopped fresh spinach

1 cup pink or green lentils, rinsed

3 cups diced tomatoes

3 cloves garlic, diced

4 cups water

2 cups vegetable stock (page 193)

1 teaspoon sea salt

¾ teaspoon fresh cracked pepper

2 teaspoons dried oregano

1 teaspoon dried thyme

1. Place everything in a slow cooker (5–6 quarts) and turn it to low. Dinner will be ready in about 6 hours.

Note: This recipe makes a lot of soup, but the consistency is loose, more soup-like than stew-like. If you want the soup to be more stew-like, reduce the water by about 1 cup.

Black Bean Soup

Black beans have long been a protein-rich staple food of many Latin cultures. This recipe is not very spicy, but if you'd like more of a kick, increase the chipotle pepper to ½ teaspoon and add some red pepper flakes. This soup is delicious served over a bowl of hot rice or with corn or brown rice chips. If you are in a hurry and do not have time to presoak and cook the black beans, have no fear! This recipe calls for organic canned beans to save you time. If you wish to soak and cook the beans first, that's great too!

SERVES 4 ◆ PREP TIME: ABOUT 1 HOUR

1 tablespoon coconut oil

1 cup chopped sweet yellow onion

1 cup chopped celery

¾ cup chopped carrots

1 jalapeño pepper, seeded and diced

2–3 cloves garlic, mashed and chopped

2 (15-ounce) cans organic black beans, rinsed and drained (or about 3½ cups cooked beans)

¾ cup chopped fresh cilantro

4 cups vegetable stock (page 193)

½ cup tomato sauce

2 tablespoons lime juice

1 tablespoon apple cider vinegar (I prefer Bragg's brand)

¼ teaspoon ground chipotle pepper

1 teaspoon cumin

Pinch of cardamom or coriander (optional)

Fresh cracked pepper and sea salt to taste

1 avocado, peeled, pitted, and sliced (optional)

1. In a Dutch oven or stock pot, heat the oil over medium to medium-high heat.

2. When the oil is hot, add the onion and sauté until soft, about 4–5 minutes. Add the celery and carrots and continue to sauté until the carrot is fork tender, about 5 minutes. Stir the jalapeño pepper, garlic, and beans into the vegetable mixture and sauté for 1 minute.

3. Add the cilantro, vegetable stock, tomato sauce, lime juice, vinegar, and seasonings (except for the pepper and salt) and stir to combine. Turn the heat down to medium-low and cook the soup for 30 minutes.

4. Transfer the soup to a blender and purée it. Return it to the soup pot and add fresh cracked pepper and salt to taste. Serve with sliced avocado, if desired.

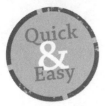

Fresh English Pea Soup

This soup delights the taste buds with its fresh peas, leeks, and tarragon. It can be served either warm or chilled. If you want to add more heat, spice up the soup with red pepper flakes. Please note that leeks are a delicate vegetable, so make sure your pot is not too hot when you cook them so they don't burn.

SERVES 4 • PREP TIME: 30 MINUTES

1 tablespoon olive oil (or coconut oil)

2 leeks, cleaned and chopped fine (about 1 heaping cup)

1 tablespoon chopped sun-dried tomatoes (optional), in oil

2 large cloves garlic, minced (about 1 tablespoon)

3 cups fresh English or petite peas

3 cups vegetable stock (page 193)

1 tablespoon fresh lemon juice

1 cup water

1 tablespoon fresh tarragon leaves

½ teaspoon fresh cracked pepper, or more to taste

Sea salt to taste

Red pepper flakes to taste

2 sliced radishes, for garnish (optional)

1. Heat a large Dutch oven or stock pot over medium heat and add the oil.

2. When the oil is hot, add the leeks and sauté them for 6–7 minutes, or until browned. Add in the sun-dried tomatoes and garlic and sauté for another 3 minutes, stirring frequently so the leeks do not stick or burn. If the leeks are cooking too quickly, reduce the heat to medium-low.

3. Add the peas, vegetable stock, lemon juice, and water, and reduce the heat to simmer. Stir in the tarragon and fresh cracked pepper and simmer for 15 minutes.

4. Turn off the heat and let the soup cool slightly. Pour half of the soup into a blender and purée it. Return the soup to the stock pot or Dutch oven and cook until it is heated through, adjusting the seasonings to taste. If serving the soup warm, dish and eat immediately. Or, chill the soup in the refrigerator before serving. Ladle the soup into individual bowls and garnish with radish slices, if you like.

Cream of Broccoli Soup

This hearty vegetable soup takes less than an hour to make and is so warm and inviting. Using parsnip purée is a tasty way to slightly thicken a soup, plus it adds more nutritional value and flavor. But if you don't have any on hand, don't worry! Replace the parsnip purée with coconut cream or, if you are even more adventurous, mashed yam!

SERVES 4   ◆   PREP TIME: ABOUT 40 MINUTES

1 tablespoon olive oil or coconut oil

1 yellow onion, chopped (about 1 cup)

5 cups chopped broccoli

3 large cloves garlic, minced

6 cups vegetable stock (page 193) (part can be water if you wish to reduce the salt content)

½ teaspoon red chili flakes

¼ teaspoon coriander

½ teaspoon fresh cracked pepper, or more or less as desired

1 tablespoon red miso

2–3 tablespoons parsnip purée (page 145), coconut cream, or cooked mashed yam

1. Heat a Dutch oven or stock pot over medium-high heat and add the oil.

2. Add in the onion and sauté it until soft, about 4 minutes. Add the broccoli and continue to sauté for 4–5 minutes, adding in a tablespoon or two of vegetable stock if the vegetables begin to stick. Stir in the garlic.

3. Reduce the heat to medium-low and add the vegetable stock, seasonings, and miso. Simmer the soup over medium-low heat for about 20 minutes, then add the parsnip purée. Cook for another 3–4 minutes, adjust the seasonings, if desired, and serve.

Creamy Butternut Squash Soup

Did you know that butternut squash and other gourds are actually fruits? Yes, they are, because they contain seeds. You may have noticed that butternut squash is my favorite kind of squash! I use it quite often in my recipes. There are many health benefits of eating butternut squash—it is low in fat and high in fiber, and it supplies a significant amount of potassium and vitamin B-6, which are good for our bones and immune systems. It also has a great flavor and can be used in a myriad of ways.

SERVES 4 ◆ PREP TIME: ABOUT 45 MINUTES

1 tablespoon coconut oil

1 cup diced onion

1 cup chopped red bell pepper

1 cup chopped fresh tomatoes

3–4 cloves garlic, minced

1 heaping tablespoon grated fresh ginger

3 cups cooked or roasted cubed butternut squash

1 cups cashew or other milk

½ cup coconut milk or coconut cream

2 cups vegetable stock (page 193)

2 teaspoons red curry paste

Lots of fresh cracked pepper

½ teaspoon sea salt

¼ teaspoon cardamom (optional)

1. In a Dutch oven or stock pot, heat the oil over medium-high heat.

2. When the oil is hot, add the onion and sauté it for 3–4 minutes, or until soft. Add the red bell pepper, tomatoes, garlic, and ginger and continue to cook for another 2–3 minutes. If the mixture begins to stick on the bottom of the pot, reduce the heat to medium. Add the butternut squash and stir to blend the vegetable mixture.

3. Add the milks, vegetable stock, red curry paste, fresh cracked pepper, salt, and cardamom. Stir well. Reduce the heat to medium-low and simmer the soup for about 30 minutes to allow the flavors to blend. If desired, transfer the soup to a blender and purée until smooth; or, if you like chunky soup, keep it as it is and serve.

Note: If you like smooth puréed soups, follow the step at the end to blend the soup. I prefer the chunks of veggies in my soup, but you can serve it either way.

Raw Avocado and Corn Soup with Cilantro Pesto

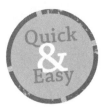

This soup, topped with the cilantro pesto, is bursting with fresh flavors and is a great dish to serve in the summer and early autumn. If you make the pesto ahead of time, this soup is a snap to make! All you will have to do to make the soup is toast the cashews and blend the ingredients—no cooking necessary. If you don't use up all the pesto on your soup, you can also eat it on top of brown rice noodles, kelp noodles, or spaghetti squash; on toasted bread; or as a topping for yams or pizza, just to name a few options. If you have an allergy to nuts, omit the cashews, and it will still be a delicious pesto!

MAKES 1 CUP OF PESTO AND 6 CUPS OF SOUP • PREP TIME: 10–15 MINUTES FOR BOTH PESTO AND SOUP

Pesto:

½ cup chopped raw cashews

1 clove garlic, minced

⅓ cup olive oil

Juice of 1–2 limes

1 large bunch cilantro, de-stemmed and washed well

2–3 tablespoons Parmesan cheese or Mock Parmesan Cheese (page 201)

Fresh cracked pepper and sea salt to taste

Soup:

3 ears fresh corn, shucked (about 3½ cups corn)

2 ripe avocados, peeled, seeded, and diced (about 1 heaping cup)

2 limes, squeezed

1–2 tablespoons fresh chopped cilantro

1½–2 tablespoons maple syrup

2 cups water

½ teaspoon sea salt

Fresh cracked pepper to taste

1 small, fresh, chopped serrano pepper

¼ teaspoon cumin

¼ teaspoon ground chipotle pepper (optional but delicious)

¼ cup raw cashews (or tofu if you have a nut allergy)

1 tablespoon apple cider vinegar

1. Toast the cashews and garlic in a small non-stick skillet over medium heat for 1–2 minutes, or until the nuts are lightly toasted and the aroma fills your nose. Remove the skillet from the heat.

2. Place the toasted nuts and garlic into a food processor and pulse until fine.

3. Add the olive oil and lime juice to the food processor and pulse until well blended. Add the cilantro and cheese and continue to pulse until the mixture is smooth. Season the mixture with salt and pepper to taste. Set aside. (The pesto can be stored in an airtight container in the refrigerator until ready to use, or for up to a week.)

4. When you're ready to make the soup, first carefully slice the corn kernels off the cobs with a sharp knife.

5. Place all the soup ingredients in a large food processor or blender and blend them until smooth. (If you use a blender, you may have too much soup to blend all at once; you may have to blend in batches and then combine.) Now you can either serve the soup immediately or place it in an airtight container and store in the refrigerator for later use. This soup stores well in the refrigerator for two to three days.

6. When ready to serve the soup, pour it into bowls and top each serving with a dollop of pesto.

Beet and Avocado Salad

Beets are good for us! The pigments in beets are called *betalains*, and they are a great source of phytonutrients. Studies have shown that the betalains called *betanin* (reddish pigment) and *vulgaxanthin* (yellow pigment) provide antioxidants, have anti-inflammatory properties, and support detoxification in the body.

SERVES 4 • PREP TIME: 30–40 MINUTES

4 medium red or yellow beets, scrubbed, peeled, and cut in half (about 2 cups)

1 ripe avocado, seeded, peeled, and chopped into bite-size pieces

10–12 cherry tomatoes, washed and cut in half

1 cup chopped Bartlett pears (or organic Gala apples)

1 cup chopped carrot

⅓ cup chopped raw cashews

1 tablespoon extra virgin olive oil

1 tablespoon balsamic vinegar

Pinch of cayenne pepper

Fresh cracked pepper and sea salt to taste

1. First, cook your beets. Steam the beet halves over hot water until they are fork tender, about 15 minutes. Set aside to cool. Chop into bite-size pieces.

2. Place the avocado, cherry tomatoes, pears or apples, and carrot in a large bowl. Add the cooled beets and cashews.

3. In a small bowl (or jar), whisk together (or shake well) the oil, vinegar, and cayenne pepper. Pour this over the vegetables and fruit and toss the salad to coat. Season with salt and pepper to taste and serve.

Note: This salad is quick and easy to make. Cook your beets ahead of time to decrease the preparation time needed to make the salad.

Warm or Cold Golden Beet and Apple Salad

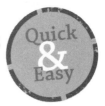

This salad can be eaten either cold or warm, but personally I love it warm! The feta cheese melts over the beets, and it is delicious. You may wish to use a dairy-free cheese, like Enjoy Your Heart mozzarella or my Mock Parmesan Cheese (see page 201).

SERVES 4 ◆ PREP TIME: 20–25 MINUTES

4 golden/yellow beets, peeled and cut into quarters

½ cup chopped walnuts, lightly toasted

1 tablespoon organic maple syrup

⅓ cup crumbled feta cheese or grated dairy-free cheese

1 large tart apple, cut into bite-size pieces

¼ cup dried cranberries

¼ cup chopped celery (optional)

1 tablespoon organic extra virgin olive oil

1 tablespoon balsamic vinegar

Sea salt and fresh cracked pepper to taste

1. Steam the quartered beets over hot water until they are fork tender, about 15 minutes.

2. While the beets are steaming, heat a small skillet over medium heat and add the chopped walnuts. Toast them lightly for about 1–3 minutes, stirring continually so they don't burn, and then remove them from the heat. Drizzle the maple syrup over the nuts and stir well to coat. Place the nuts in a large salad bowl.

3. When the beets are fork tender, cool them slightly, chop them into bite-size pieces, and add them to the salad bowl. Add the feta cheese, apple, cranberries, and celery and toss them together. If the beets are still warm, the cheese will likely melt a bit. This is a good thing!

4. In a small bowl (or jar), combine the olive oil and balsamic vinegar and whisk to fully incorporate (or shake vigorously). Pour the mixture over the salad ingredients and stir to blend the flavors together. If you want more dressing, double the recommended amounts.

Black-Eyed Pea Salad

I never ate black-eyed peas as a child, but when I finally tried them, I loved them! One cup of the peas provides 4.5 grams of protein and less than 1 gram of fat. One cup of them contains about 160 calories. They are a good source of fiber and a rich source of potassium, zinc, and vitamin C. Eat this salad as is, or serve it over cooked quinoa or fresh greens from the garden.

SERVES 4 • PREP TIME: ABOUT 1 HOUR, PLUS SOAKING AND COOKING TIME FOR THE BEANS

1 cup dry or 3 cups cooked black-eyed peas

1 cup fresh green beans, ends removed

1 ripe avocado, peeled, seeded, and diced

1 medium jalapeño, seeded and finely chopped (about 2 tablespoons)

1 large red bell pepper, chopped (about 1 cup)

2 tablespoons olive oil

2 tablespoons GF teriyaki sauce (such as Annie Chun's brand)

1 tablespoon red wine vinegar

1 tablespoon fresh lemon juice

Fresh cracked pepper and sea salt to taste

1. If you are using black-eyed peas that are already cooked, skip to step 2. If you are starting with dry beans, sort the beans and remove any clumps of dirt, and then wash well to remove any dirt. Place the beans in a large bowl, cover them with water, and soak them for at least 8 hours, or overnight. Drain the beans and rinse them well. Place the beans in a stock pot and add enough water to cover them, then add a pinch of salt. Bring the water to a boil, then reduce the heat to medium-low (so they simmer gently) and cook until tender, about 45 minutes. Let the beans cool completely and then drain.

2. Steam the green beans over hot water until fork tender, about 4–5 minutes, then let them cool completely. Chop the green beans into bite-size pieces.

3. Put the peas, green beans, avocado, jalapeño pepper, and red bell pepper in a large bowl and toss them to combine.

4. In a small bowl (or jar), combine the olive oil, teriyaki sauce, vinegar, and lemon juice. Whisk well (or shake vigorously) to fully emulsify the ingredients and then pour this dressing over the salad. Season the salad with fresh cracked pepper and salt to taste and serve.

Broccoli Salad with Sesame Tahini and Lime Dressing

This colorful and flavorful salad is easy to make and full of healthy ingredients. The sesame tahini and lime dressing is wonderful on this salad, and if you don't use it all up on the salad, it's great drizzled over roasted vegetables or baked garnet yams. You can make the dressing ahead of time and store it in an airtight container in the fridge to cut down on the preparation time for this salad. Or, if you want to try a different flavor on the broccoli salad, try it with the Almond Curry Dressing found on page 187.

MAKES 1 CUP OF DRESSING AND 4 SERVINGS OF SALAD • PREP TIME: LESS THAN 20 MINUTES

Sesame Tahini and Lime Dressing:

3 teaspoons mustard

3 tablespoons sesame tahini

3 tablespoons coconut cream (or canned coconut milk, full fat)

3 tablespoons grapeseed oil

4 tablespoons freshly squeezed lime juice

2 teaspoons kelp granules (optional)

½ teaspoon sea salt, plus more to taste

Fresh cracked pepper to taste

Salad:

4 cups chopped broccoli (from about 2 heads of broccoli)

½ cup peeled and grated jicama

¼ cup chopped raw walnuts

⅓ cup dried cherries, chopped

⅓ cup mung bean sprouts (or other sprouts, if desired)

1 medium red bell pepper, chopped (about ½ cup)

3 tablespoons minced red onion

1 tablespoon chopped Anaheim pepper (optional)

1. Place all of the dressing ingredients into a blender and whirl to fully incorporate. Season the dressing to taste with salt and pepper. Set the dressing aside or store it in an airtight container in the refrigerator for later use.

2. Put all of the salad ingredients into a large bowl and drizzle with about ½ cup of the dressing. Toss the salad well and serve.

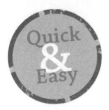

English Pea Salad

If you can't find English peas, don't sweat it. I have made this salad with fresh peas from the market, and I have friends who have made it with peas from their gardens! The seasonings in this salad are very basic, but they offer a lovely, light Asian flavor. This salad is so delicious, you may want to double the recipe. The salad keeps well in the fridge for several days and is great to pack in school lunches, for a quick pick-me-up snack in the middle of the afternoon, or as a topping for a green salad.

SERVES 4 ◆ PREP TIME: ABOUT 15 MINUTES

1 cup English peas

1 cup halved cherry tomatoes

1 cup snow peas, strings and tips removed, sliced in half

½ cup chopped carrot

2 teaspoons sesame oil

1 tablespoon tamari sauce

Sea salt and fresh cracked pepper to taste

Sesame seeds, for garnish (optional)

1. Steam the English peas over hot water for 3–4 minutes. Remove them from the steamer and set them aside.

2. Put the chopped vegetables in a large bowl and add the steamed peas.

3. In a small bowl (or jar), combine the sesame oil and tamari sauce and whisk well to fully incorporate (or shake well). Pour the dressing over the salad and toss well to coat. Season with salt and pepper to taste. If desired, sprinkle sesame seeds on top of the salad for extra texture.

Strawberry Salad with Mint Dressing and Greens

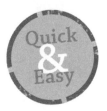

This is a quintessential spring or summer salad—a great dish to bring to an outdoor party! The greens (arugula and butter lettuce) are delightful paired with the purple cabbage, raw cashews, strawberries, and fresh mint. The addition of gorgonzola cheese is the icing on the cake. If you are dairy-free, try a sprinkling of kelp flakes, sunflower seeds, or Mock Parmesan Cheese (page 201) instead.

SERVES 4 • PREP TIME: ABOUT 15 MINUTES

½ cup shredded purple cabbage

1 cup arugula

1 large head butter lettuce, cut into bite-size pieces

½ cup chopped Medjool dates

¼ cup raw cashews

2 cups sliced fresh strawberries

¼ cup gorgonzola cheese (optional)

½ cup vegan sour cream (see Mock Sour Cream, page 201)

2 tablespoons freshly squeezed orange juice

1 tablespoon chopped fresh mint

Sea salt and fresh cracked pepper to taste

Mint leaves, for garnish

1. Put the cabbage, arugula, lettuce, dates, cashews, strawberries, and cheese in a large bowl and toss to combine.

2. In a small bowl, combine the sour cream, orange juice, mint, and salt and pepper to taste.

3. If you plan to serve the entire salad and not have any leftovers, toss the dressing with the salad ingredients. If you think there will be leftover salad, then serve the dressing on the side so the leftovers won't wilt. Garnish the salad with fresh mint leaves before serving.

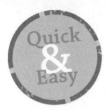

Delicious Apple-Kale Slaw

The health benefits of kale are endless! Kale has been called the healthiest vegetable on the planet because it is incredibly high in vitamins, minerals, phytonutrients, and antioxidants. When I make this slaw, I don't pour the dressing over the entire salad. I prefer to drizzle the dressing over individual servings so that the salad isn't totally saturated with the dressing—but it is up to your personal preference!

SERVES 4 TO 6 ● PREP TIME: ABOUT 10 MINUTES

Vegetables:

1 large bunch Tuscan kale, finely chopped (about 4 cups)

1¼ cup grated red cabbage (or green cabbage)

1–2 tart red apples (such as Cripps Pink), grated (about 1 cup)

½ cup grated carrot

½ cup finely chopped raw walnuts

Dressing:

¾ cup freshly squeezed orange juice

¼ cup organic olive oil

¼ teaspoon sea salt

1 teaspoon Bragg's Organic Sprinkle (optional) or a pinch of fresh rosemary and fresh cracked pepper

1. Place the chopped kale in a large bowl. Add the cabbage, apple, carrots, and walnuts to the bowl. Toss the ingredients to combine.

2. Place the dressing ingredients in a small bowl (or jar) and whisk well (or shake vigorously), until the mixture is fully combined.

3. To serve as slaw, pour the dressing over the entire salad and toss to combine. Or, place one serving of the salad in a bowl or plate and drizzle dressing over the top. Store the unused salad in an airtight container in the fridge. Store the dressing in an airtight container (or in the jar you mixed it in) in the fridge. Both will keep for a few days.

Jicama and Fruit Slaw

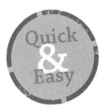

Jicama is such an underrated vegetable. I think the reason is that many people are unfamiliar with jicama and how to use it in recipes. Jicama is versatile—it has a lovely texture but not an over-powering flavor—which makes it so easy to add to recipes. To go with the jicama, this recipe calls for apples, oranges, and pears, but you can add other fruits or vegetables as well, such as nectarines, cabbage, or dried cranberries, to name just a few. The flavors of cumin, mint, and jalapeño really spice this recipe up and give it some punch!

MAKES ABOUT 6 CUPS • PREP TIME: ABOUT 30 MINUTES

2 tablespoons orange juice

¼ cup lime juice

¼ cup olive oil

½ teaspoon sea salt

2 tablespoons chopped fresh mint

¼ cup chopped fresh basil

½ teaspoon ground cumin

2½ cups grated jicama

1 large apple (Granny Smith or Gala work well), grated

2 avocados, peeled, seeded, and chopped into bite-size pieces

1 small pear, washed and diced

1 orange, peeled, pith removed, and sectioned

1 small jalapeño pepper, washed, seeds removed, and finely diced (about 1 tablespoon)

Fresh basil or mint leaves, for garnish (optional)

1. Place the orange juice, lime juice, olive oil, salt, mint, basil, and cumin in a blender and whirl to fully incorporate the ingredients. Set the mixture aside.

2. In a large bowl, combine the jicama, apple, avocado, pear, orange, and jalapeño pepper.

3. Pour the dressing over the top of the salad and toss it well. Put the salad in the refrigerator and let it rest for up to 30 minutes to allow the flavors to blend. Dish out servings and garnish with fresh mint or basil leaves, if desired.

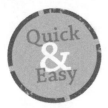

Edamame and Quinoa Salad

This easy-to-make salad can be served warm or cold. It's a great dish to pack up for the kids to eat at school because it provides a great source of protein and is light and flavorful. This salad is also delicious served in a lettuce wrap.

SERVES 4 • PREP TIME: 20–25 MINUTES

1 cup dry quinoa, thoroughly rinsed and drained

2 cups vegetable stock (page 193)

2 cups shelled edamame

½ cup chopped fire-roasted bell peppers (any peppers will do, but fire-roasted peppers add more flavor)

3 tablespoons lemon juice, or more if desired

2 tablespoons olive oil

¼–½ teaspoon sea salt

1 tablespoon fresh tarragon (or fresh mint)

Lemon zest (optional)

1 tablespoon organic maple syrup

Fresh cracked pepper to taste

Additional tarragon or lemon zest, for garnish (optional)

1. Place the quinoa and vegetable stock in a 2-quart saucepan, cover, and bring to a boil over medium-high heat. When the mixture has reached a boil, reduce the heat to low, and simmer until the liquid is nearly absorbed, about 10 minutes.

2. Add the edamame to the quinoa, cover, and cook for another 5–6 minutes, or until the liquid has been absorbed and the quinoa is light and fluffy. Mix in the peppers.

3. Place the lemon juice, olive oil, salt, tarragon, lemon zest, and syrup in a small bowl (or jar). Whisk well (or shake vigorously) for 30 seconds. Pour the liquid ingredients over the quinoa and edamame mixture. Toss to mix. Season with fresh cracked pepper to taste. Serve the salad warm, or place it in the refrigerator to chill. When ready to serve the salad, garnish it with tarragon or lemon zest, if desired.

Quinoa Tabouli Salad

I used to eat traditional tabouli salad when I was younger, which is made from cracked wheat/bulger. When I started eating gluten-free, I switched to using quinoa instead, and I love it! This salad is perfect to take along to work for lunch, share at a potluck, or serve as a dinner salad alongside a bowl of soup.

SERVES 4 ◆ PREP TIME: 35 MINUTES, INCLUDING MARINATING

2 cups cooked quinoa

¼ cup chopped red, yellow, or green bell pepper

½ cup grated carrot

1 cup diced Persian seedless cucumbers (or other varieties)

¼ cup minced red onion

1 cup chopped tomato

2 teaspoons minced garlic

1 tablespoon olive oil

3 tablespoons lemon juice

⅓ cup finely chopped fresh parsley

1 teaspoon dried spearmint leaves (or 2 tablespoons fresh)

Sea salt and fresh cracked pepper to taste

1. Place the quinoa and all of the vegetables in a large serving bowl.

2. Put the oil, lemon juice, parsley, spearmint, salt, and pepper in a small bowl (or jar) and whisk well (or shake vigorously) to combine. Pour the dressing over the entire salad and toss to combine.

3. Let the salad sit in the refrigerator for up to 30 minutes to marinate. Serve immediately.

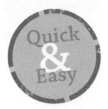

Asian Brown Rice Salad

This salad is packed with protein and complex carbs—it is truly a hearty meal! If you are allergic to soy or are avoiding it, leave out the edamame and replace it with cooked kidney beans. If you have a nut allergy, simply leave out the cashews. Pineapple adds a nice sweetness to this salad, and the enzymes in pineapple aid digestion. But don't worry if you don't have any pineapple in the house to use—the salad still tastes great without it!

SERVES 4 ◆ PREP TIME: 10–15 MINUTES

Salad:

1 cup raw cashews

1 tablespoon honey (or brown rice syrup)

½ teaspoon curry powder

3 cups cooked short-grain brown rice

1 cup bean sprouts

1 cup drained and sliced water chestnuts

¾ cup diced celery

½ cup snow peas, sliced (optional)

1 cup fresh pineapple chunks, cut into bite-size pieces

1 cup cooked edamame, shelled

⅓ cup raisins

¼ cup chopped green or red bell pepper

2 tablespoons sesame seeds

Dressing:

¼ teaspoon sea salt (I prefer Himalayan salt)

2 tablespoons rice vinegar

⅛ cup GF tamari sauce

¼ cup sesame tahini

¼ cup olive oil

⅛ cup freshly squeezed lime juice

Sea salt and fresh cracked pepper to taste

1. Heat a small skillet over medium-high heat and add the cashews. Lightly toast the nuts, stirring frequently. When the nuts are warm and slightly browned, remove from the heat and drizzle the honey over the top. Then sprinkle on the curry powder and stir to blend together. Set the cashews aside.

2. Put the rest of the salad ingredients together in a large bowl, add the toasted cashews, and toss all of the ingredients to distribute evenly.

3. In a small bowl (or jar), combine all of the dressing ingredients (except for the salt and pepper) and whisk well (or shake vigorously). When fully emulsified, pour the dressing over the salad and toss to coat well. Season with salt and fresh cracked pepper to taste. Serve immediately.

Sesame Noodle Salad

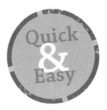

This salad is delicious with either kelp noodles or rice noodles. Kelp noodles are allergen-free, require no cooking, and have a lovely crunch. They are easy to prepare—just wash, chop, and toss them into the salad bowl. If you use rice noodles, the salad will turn out a bit heartier. Be sure not to overcook the rice noodles: they should be al dente!

SERVES 4 ◆ PREP TIME: LESS THAN 30 MINUTES

Salad:

8 ounces rice noodles or kelp noodles

10 green onions/scallions, chopped (about ½ cup)

1 cup bean sprouts, optional

½ cup chopped fresh cilantro

Additional fresh cilantro, for garnish

2 tablespoons sesame seeds, for garnish

Dressing:

½–1 teaspoon toasted sesame oil

1 tablespoon GF tamari sauce

2 tablespoons peanut butter (or sesame tahini)

1 tablespoon olive oil

1 tablespoon honey

1 teaspoon minced garlic (optional)

1 teaspoon ground ginger

1. If you are using rice noodles, cook them according to the directions on the package, rinse them in cold water, and drain the water. Place in a large bowl. If you are using kelp noodles, rinse them well, chop them and place them in a large bowl.

2. Add the green onions, bean sprouts, and cilantro.

3. Combine the dressing ingredients in a small bowl (or jar), whisk well (or shake vigorously) to combine, and pour it over the top of the noodles and vegetables. Toss in the dressing well to cover all of the noodles and serve the salad cold. Garnish the salad with fresh cilantro and sesame seeds.

Main Dishes

Tempeh and Veggie Bourgignon

This is a fabulous recipe! The marinated tempeh takes on the rich flavor of the wine and mushrooms and bursts with flavor. You can marinate the tempeh an hour before you want to start cooking, or marinate the tempeh up to two days ahead of time so it's ready to go. I love to serve this recipe over red or brown rice, but you could also serve it like a stroganoff over gluten-free noodles or polenta—your kids will love it!

SERVES 4 • PREP TIME: ABOUT 90 MINUTES

¾ cup chopped red onion

1 (8-ounce) package GF tempeh, cut into 1-inch cubes

½ cup chopped carrot

1 cup fingerling potatoes (small yellow potatoes)

2 cloves garlic, finely chopped

1½ cups medium-bodied red wine (such as Cabernet)

¾ cup vegetable stock (page 193)

½ teaspoon Herbes de Provence

¼ teaspoon tarragon (optional)

2 tablespoons olive oil

1 tablespoon balsamic vinegar

3 tablespoons organic tomato paste

3 cups chopped cremini or portobello mushrooms

¼ cup chopped fresh parsley

Sea salt and fresh cracked pepper to taste

1. In a large bowl, combine the onion, tempeh, carrots, potatoes, garlic, wine, vegetable stock, and spices. Set this mixture aside to marinate for an hour (or up to two days prior to use).

2. Strain all of the vegetables and tempeh out of the wine mixture, but also retain the marinade, as it will be used later.

3. Heat a large skillet or Dutch oven to medium-high heat and put in 1 tablespoon of the olive oil.

4. When the oil is hot, add the tempeh and vegetables to the skillet or Dutch oven and sauté for 10 minutes. Add in the balsamic vinegar and stir to combine. Add in the tomato paste and continue stirring for 1–2 minutes.

5. Add the marinade and mushrooms to the skillet or Dutch oven, then reduce the heat to medium-low, and cover. Let it simmer for 30 minutes, checking the pan every 10 minutes to see if the liquid has been absorbed. If the vegetables are getting dry, add a splash of vegetable stock to keep them just barely covered. You may want to poke the vegetables down into the marinade so they cook thoroughly.

6. Once the carrots and potatoes are fork tender, add the parsley and season with the salt and fresh cracked pepper to taste. If your vegetables are cut into larger pieces, they may require a few extra minutes of cooking time to ensure they are done. Serve immediately.

Vegetarian Shepherd's Pie

I love the flavors of this shepherd's pie. Though there is red curry paste in the recipe, it is very mild. I developed this recipe for the family, so I went light with the spices; you can add more heat to the dish, if you like, by adding hot sauce or cayenne pepper. If you have made the Cajun Smashed Sweet Potatoes (page 143) or Cauliflower Mashed "Potatoes" (page 144), they both make a tasty substitution for the mashed potatoes.

SERVES 4 • PREP TIME: 1½ HOURS (IF YOU USE PRE-MADE MASHED POTATOES, PREP TIME WILL BE ABOUT 40 MINUTES LESS)

4 medium Yukon gold potatoes, peeled and quartered

¾ cup reserved potato water

Sea salt and fresh cracked pepper to taste

1 tablespoon olive oil

1 cup chopped onions

¾ cup chopped carrots

3 cups chopped broccoli

¼–½ cup vegetable stock (page 193)

1 cup peas

1 cup sprouted organic tofu, cut into small bite-size pieces

2 cloves garlic, chopped

1 cup sliced cremini or other mushrooms

1 cup organic canned coconut milk

1 tablespoon red curry paste

½ teaspoon cumin

¼ teaspoon coriander

1 tablespoon arrowroot powder

Sea salt and fresh cracked pepper to taste

1. Bring a large pot of water to boil and drop in the peeled, quarter potatoes. Reduce the heat to medium or medium-low and simmer until the potatoes are fork tender, about 40 minutes.

2. Drain the potatoes over a bowl so you can reserve the water. Mash the potatoes with ¾ cup of the reserved water (you can either discard the rest of the reserved potato water or keep it for soup). Season with salt and pepper to taste. Set the potatoes aside.

3. Preheat the oven to 350°F.

4. Heat a large skillet or Dutch oven over medium-high heat and add the olive oil.

5. When the oil is hot, add the onion and sauté for a few minutes, or until soft. Add the carrots and broccoli and continue to sauté for 3–4 minutes. If the vegetables begin to stick to the bottom of the skillet or Dutch oven, add a little bit of the vegetable stock and continue cooking. Add in the vegetable stock, peas, tofu, garlic, and mushrooms and continue to sauté for another 2–3 minutes.

6. Add in the coconut milk, red curry paste, cumin, and coriander. Reduce the heat to medium-low and add the arrowroot powder into the simmering vegetables and sauce and quickly whisk the mixture to fully incorporate the arrowroot powder. The mixture should begin to thicken. If it does not thicken, you will need to turn the heat up to medium-high until the

mixture is boiling and it thickens. Remove it from the heat, and season with salt and pepper to taste.

7. Carefully pour the vegetables and sauce into a 9 × 9-inch baking dish. Layer the mashed potatoes over the top of the vegetable mixture, making sure to cover the entire top of the dish. Season with salt and pepper.

8. Bake uncovered in a 350°F oven for about 45 minutes, or until the mixture is bubbling at the edges. Remove the pan from the oven. Turn the oven to broil and raise the oven rack to the top shelf. Put the baking dish on the top shelf and broil for about 1–2 minutes to brown the top of the casserole. Remove it from the oven, let it sit for 5 minutes to cool slightly, and serve.

Bean and Corn Patties with Greens

These patties are made with garbanzo beans, which are chock-full of protein. The Herbes de Provence and fire-roasted red or yellow bell peppers offer lovely flavors and, paired with the greens, a complete meal. I like to wilt some spinach lightly to serve the patties over, but you can also use fresh greens, such as baby arugula. I like to drizzle a bit of lemon juice and olive oil over the top of the patties and greens, and then add some fresh cracked pepper to taste.

MAKES 8 PATTIES • PREP TIME: 45–50 MINUTES

2 cups cooked garbanzo beans, drained (see directions below)

1 teaspoon plus 1–2 tablespoons coconut oil, separated

⅓ cups finely chopped shallots (or sweet yellow onion)

1½ cups fresh organic, non-GMO corn, husked (or frozen if fresh is not available)

¼ teaspoon Herbes de Provence (or dried thyme)

1 tablespoon chopped fresh parsley

1 teaspoon sea salt

Fresh cracked pepper to taste (up to ½ teaspoon)

½ cup crushed rice chips or crackers (or GF breadcrumbs)

4 tablespoons cornmeal

2 tablespoons chopped fire-roasted red or yellow bell peppers

Spinach, arugula, or other greens, raw or steamed

1. If you are using dried garbanzo beans, soak them in water overnight. Drain off the water they were soaked in several times, until the water runs clear. In a large pot, cover the beans with water and simmer over low heat until done, checking for doneness after 30 minutes. Drain the beans again and put 2 cups of the cooked beans into a food processor. Set it aside.

2. Heat a small skillet over medium-high heat and add 1 teaspoon of the oil.

3. When the oil is hot, add in the shallots and cook for 1 minute, stirring constantly. Add in the corn and continue to sauté for another 2–3 minutes. Add the Herbes de Provence, parsley, salt, and pepper. Remove the skillet from the heat and set it aside.

4. Add the crushed rice crackers or bread crumbs to the food processor, as well as the cornmeal and bell peppers. Pulse this mixture several times, until it begins to blend together. Add in the corn and shallot mixture, pulsing 10–12 times, or until the mixture is a consistency that is easy to form into patties. Don't pulse so much that it turns to mush!

5. With clean hands, form the mixture into 8 patties, each about 3 inches around and 1 inch thick.

6. Heat a large skillet over medium heat and add in some of the remaining oil, about ½ tablespoon. Put 4 of the patties in the skillet. Cook them for about 5 minutes on each side, checking often. You want the patties to be cooked through and golden brown; if they are cooking too quickly or burning, adjust the heat as needed. Remove the patties when they are done, and repeat the cooking process for the remaining 4 patties.

7. Serve the patties over lightly wilted spinach, fresh arugula, or other greens. The patties will last a few days in the refrigerator and, if desired, can be frozen in a ziplock plastic bag for up to a month.

Quinoa Burgers

These are delicious burgers that the kids will love! The patties tend to be a bit crumbly and don't always stay together, so I recommend serving them on top of fresh greens with sprouts, avocado, and tomato. You can serve them on GF buns, if you prefer. They may fall apart, but your family will scramble to eat all of the pieces, I guarantee you! My favorite brand of ground vegetable protein is Helen's Kitchen because it is organic and GMO-free. Look for it at your local health-food store or buy it online. It is worth having in the refrigerator!

MAKES 5 PATTIES ♦ PREP TIME: 30–40 MINUTES

1 teaspoon chia seeds whisked with 2 tablespoons water

1 tablespoon coconut oil

1 cup finely chopped red onion

½ cup diced shiitake mushrooms

1 (12-ounce) package vegetable protein crumbles

2 cloves garlic, minced

¼ cup GF oats

1 cup cooked organic red quinoa

1 teaspoon Dijon mustard

2 tablespoons non-dairy cream cheese (optional)

1 egg, beaten well

2 teaspoons smoked paprika

2 tablespoons finely chopped fresh parsley

Coconut oil spray for cooking

1. Place the chia seeds in a small bowl and add the water. Whisk together well and set the mixture aside to allow it to gel for 5–6 minutes.

2. In a large skillet, heat the oil over medium heat and add the onion. Sauté until soft, about 4 minutes. Add the mushrooms and continue to sauté for another 2–3 minutes. Add the vegetable protein crumbles, garlic, oats, and quinoa and stir to incorporate. Add the mustard, cream cheese, egg, paprika, and parsley, and the chia seed mixture, and stir together well. Remove the skillet from heat and set it aside.

3. Heat a non-stick skillet over low heat (I set my burner to 3, which is low) and lightly spray the pan with coconut oil. Put a half-cup of the quinoa mixture into the heated pan. Press lightly on the mixture, not making the patty too flat. The patty will hold up better if you keep it thick. Cook for 4 minutes over medium-low heat and then carefully flip it over. Cook it on the other side for another 4 minutes, then carefully transfer the patty to a serving dish. Continue to cook all of the burgers using the same process. If needed, you can keep them warm in a 200°F oven until you have cooked them all.

Quinoa and Veggie Burgers

Kale is one of the healthiest vegetables on the planet. I've heard it called the Queen of the Greens! One cup of chopped kale contains 33 calories and 9 percent of the daily value of calcium, 206 percent of vitamin A, 134 percent of vitamin C, and a whopping 684 percent of vitamin K. It is also a good source of minerals copper, potassium, iron, manganese, and phosphorus.

Kale's health benefits are due to the high concentration of antioxidant vitamins A, C, and K and sulphur-containing phytonutrients. I added quinoa to this burger to add protein and a nutty flavor. These burgers can be served in a lettuce wrap, on a GF bun, over greens, or by themselves topped with hummus and fresh tomato.

SERVES 4 ● PREP TIME: ABOUT 30 MINUTES

¾ cup water

½ cup quinoa, rinsed

1 cup chopped kale

1 cup finely chopped onion

1 cup thinly sliced cremini mushrooms

¼ cup roasted red bell peppers

1 medium carrot, chopped

½–¾ cup rice cracker crumbs (start with ½ cup and add more if needed)

1 large egg, beaten

2 tablespoons lemon juice, freshly squeezed if possible

½ teaspoon chili powder

Sea salt and fresh cracked pepper to taste

2 tablespoons coconut oil

1. Heat the water to boil in a 2-quart sauce pan and add the quinoa. Cover the pan and reduce the heat to medium-low. Simmer for 13–14 minutes, or until the liquid has been absorbed. Remove the pan from the heat and set it aside.

2. Put all the ingredients (except the oil) into the food processor and pulse until mixture is just combined and begins to stick together. Remove the mixture from the food processor and form it into burger-size patties. This recipe should make 4 patties.

3. Heat a large skillet over medium-high heat and add 1 tablespoon of the oil. When the oil is hot, place the patties into the skillet and cook on each side about 4 minutes, or until browned, then reduce the heat to medium-low, cover the pan, and cook until heated through, another 5 minutes or so. Serve immediately.

Mu Shu Wraps, Vegetarian-Style

This is a fun recipe to prepare with kids! There are so many options for what to use as wraps: I like to use romaine lettuce leaves, but you can also try rice paper wraps, hemp or brown rice tortillas, or butter leaf lettuce. Traditionally, hoisin sauce is used in the wraps, but it contains wheat, so this version calls for a chili sauce. I would recommend a Vietnamese- or Thai-style chili sauce, which can be purchased at your local market.

SERVES 4 ◆ PREP TIME: ABOUT 30–40 MINUTES

Filling:

1 cup dried shiitake mushrooms

1 cup thinly sliced red onion

2 tablespoons thinly sliced fresh ginger

3 cloves garlic, minced

3 cups finely chopped or grated green cabbage

1½ cups grated carrots

1 cup grated zucchini

3 green onions/scallions, sliced lengthwise

1 cup snow peas, sliced lengthwise into several pieces

2 eggs, beaten

1 teaspoon GF tamari sauce

1 teaspoon sesame oil

1 teaspoon plus 2 teaspoons coconut oil, separated

Sesame seeds, if desired

Kelp granules, sea salt, and fresh cracked pepper to taste, if desired

Sauce:

water (retained from mushrooms) or vegetable stock (page 193)

2 teaspoons tamari sauce

2 teaspoons sesame oil

1 tablespoon rice wine vinegar

1 teaspoon brown rice syrup or maple syrup

1 tablespoon tamarind sauce (optional)

2 teaspoons arrowroot powder

For the Wraps:

Rice paper (egg roll wraps); or brown rice, hemp, or other GF tortilla; or romaine or butter lettuce leaves

Thai-style chili sauce, if desired

1. Place the dried shiitakes in a small bowl and add just enough water to cover. Let the mushrooms soak for 20–30 minutes, then drain them, reserving the water for the sauce. Slice the mushrooms thinly.

2. To make the filling, prepare the onion, ginger, garlic, cabbage, carrots, zucchini, green onions, and snow peas. Place them in separate small bowls and set aside.

3. To prepare the sauce, combine the water or stock, tamari, sesame oil, vinegar, syrup, and tamarind sauce in a small saucepan. Heat these ingredients over medium heat and then whisk in the arrowroot powder, stirring constantly, so it doesn't lump. Remove the sauce from the heat when it thickens and begins to bubble. Set it aside.

4. To prepare the egg mixture for the filling, whisk the beaten eggs with the 1 teaspoon tamari sauce and 1 teaspoon sesame oil. Heat a wok or large skillet to medium-high and put in the 1 teaspoon of coconut oil. When the oil is hot, add the egg mixture and swirl it around in the pan so it forms a thin, round layer, as though you are starting to cook an omelet. Cook the egg for one minute, then flip it over and continue to cook it for 1 more minute. Remove the egg from the pan and cool it on a plate. When the egg is cool, slice it into thin strips and set aside.

5. Wipe any leftover egg scraps from the wok or skillet and add the 2 teaspoons of coconut oil. Heat the pan to medium-high heat.

6. When hot, add the onion and ginger and sauté for 3–4 minutes, then add the mushrooms, garlic, cabbage, carrots, zucchini, and green onions and snow peas and continue to sauté for 5–6 minutes, or until the vegetables are al dente.

7. Add the sauce to the vegetables and the sesame seeds, if desired, and stir well to incorporate. Add the egg slices and stir them into the mixture. Continue to cook the mixture until the sauce has thickened and the vegetables are cooked. Season with kelp granules, salt, and fresh cracked pepper, if desired.

8. It's fun to let your family or guests create their own wraps. If you're using rice paper or tortillas as your wraps, heat them up. If you're using lettuce leaves as wraps, wash and dry them, and place them on a plate. Serve the Mu Shu veggies on a large platter and have the chili sauce at hand for your family to top their wraps with, if desired.

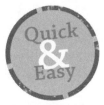

Stir-Fried Vegetables and Rice

Edamame provides the protein in this dish, but if you prefer tofu, just substitute it, using the same amount. I love to use a combination of red and black rice because it has more flavor than brown rice alone, but don't make a special trip to the market; any short- or long-grain brown rice will work nicely in this recipe. I don't recommend white rice because it's high in simple carbs and doesn't contain much nutrition. When I make this recipe, I use quite a lot of red pepper flakes to make the dish spicy, but if you have kids that are not crazy about spicy foods, you don't have to add them.

SERVES 4 ◆ PREP TIME: ABOUT 30 MINUTES

2 eggs

1 teaspoon plus 2 tablespoons tamari sauce, separated

1 teaspoon toasted sesame oil

1 tablespoon coconut oil

1 cup chopped red cabbage

1 cup diced yellow onion

1 teaspoon minced fresh ginger

2 cloves garlic, diced

¾ cup snow peas, strings removed and cut in half diagonally

1 cup cremini mushrooms, cleaned, stems removed, and sliced in half

½ cup shelled edamame (or tofu)

3 tablespoons green onions/scallions

Crushed red pepper (optional)

2 cups cooked red or brown rice, or a combination

Sea salt and fresh cracked pepper to taste

Kelp granules, if desired

1. In a small bowl, beat the eggs with 1 teaspoon tamari sauce.

2. Heat the sesame oil in a large wok or skillet over medium heat. When the oil is hot, put in the egg mixture and scramble the eggs, stirring frequently, for 2–3 minutes, or until the egg is cooked. Remove the eggs from the heat and set aside.

3. Clean excess egg scraps from the pan and then return the wok or skillet to the heat and add the coconut oil. Heat the pan to medium-high and add the cabbage and yellow onion. Cook until onion is soft, about 4 minutes. Add the ginger, garlic, snow peas, and mushrooms and continue sautéing for 4–5 minutes.

4. Add the scrambled egg, edamame, remaining 2 tablespoons tamari sauce, green onions, and crushed red pepper. Reduce the heat to low and continue to cook until the mixture is heated through, about 3 minutes.

5. Add the cooked rice to the mixture and stir together well. Continue cooking until the dish is heated through. Season with salt and pepper to taste, and, if desired, kelp granules.

Kimchi or Sauerkraut and Veggies with Noodles

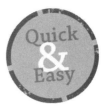

What's the difference between kimchi and sauerkraut? Kimchi is pickled vegetables and sauerkraut is fermented cabbage. Both foods offer health benefits: fermented foods help keep our gut flora healthy and cabbage is high in vitamins A and C. Cabbage is also a rich source of phytonutrients and adds wonderful flavor to foods. I created this recipe because I love kelp noodles and veggies together. This dish is great for busy nights because it's a complete meal and you can prepare it all in one pan for easy clean up.

SERVES 4 ◆ PREP TIME: LESS THAN 30 MINUTES

1 (8-ounce) package tempeh (optional)

1 (12-ounce) package kelp noodles or Pad Thai rice noodles (about 1½ cups)

1 tablespoon coconut oil

1 cup chopped red onion

1 cup chopped green beans

3 cups chopped savoy cabbage

1½ cups chopped baby bok choy

1 cup snow peas, strings and ends removed, chopped

1 tablespoon grated fresh ginger

¼ cup cilantro (optional)

1 cup curried kimchi or sauerkraut

1 teaspoon sea salt

Fresh cracked pepper to taste

1. If using tempeh, cut it into chunks and place it in a steamer on the stove. Steam for 15 minutes, or until soft. Remove from heat and set aside.

2. If using kelp noodles, rinse them. If you are using Pad Thai rice noodles, cook them according to the directions on the package, remove them from the heat, and rinse them. Chop the kelp or rice noodles into bite-size pieces.

3. Heat a large Dutch oven, wok, or skillet to medium heat and add the oil. When the oil is hot, add the onion and sauté for 4 minutes. Add in the green beans, cabbage, bok choy, and snow peas and continue to sauté for another 3 minutes.

4. Add the ginger, cilantro, kimchi or sauerkraut, and cooked tempeh to the vegetables and sauté for another 3–4 minutes, stirring constantly.

5. Put the prepared noodles into the vegetable mixture and stir to combine, until the noodles are heated through.

6. Season with the salt and fresh cracked pepper to taste. Serve immediately.

Note: I used curry or juniper berries in my sauerkraut recipe, which adds its own unique flavor to the veggie dish. If you are using an unflavored kimchi or sauerkraut, season it to taste with salt and fresh cracked pepper before using.

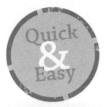

Veggie Stir-Fry with Peanut Sauce

The peanut sauce in this recipe is a real show-stopper! It is so sweet and spicy, and it can easily be made allergen-free by using sunflower seed butter in place of the peanut butter. Stir-fry, like soup, is a great way to use up a variety of vegetables, so feel free to adjust the recipe depending on what you have. I have suggested a tasty blend of veggies in this recipe, but you can use any combination of veggies you like—you will want to use 7–8 cups of veggies maximum for this recipe. What's in your refrigerator today?

SERVES 4   ●   PREP TIME: LESS THAN 20 MINUTES

Sauce:

1 cup creamy peanut butter (or sunflower seed butter)

2 tablespoons chopped fresh cilantro

1 teaspoon minced garlic

Large pinch of red pepper flakes

2 tablespoons honey or brown rice syrup

1 cup hot water

Stir-Fry:

1 tablespoon coconut oil

1 cup chopped onion

2 cups chopped broccoli

1 cup chopped cauliflower

3 cups chopped kale

2–3 cloves garlic, minced

Cooked quinoa, red rice, or pasta

1. Place all of the ingredients for the sauce into a food processor and pulse until smooth and creamy. Pour the sauce into a serving dish and set it aside.

2. Heat a large skillet over medium heat and add the oil. When the oil is hot, add the onion and sauté it, stirring frequently, about 4–5 minutes, or until soft. Add in the broccoli, cauliflower, and kale and continue to sauté for another 4–5 minutes. Add the garlic and sauté for another minute. Continue to stir the mixture occasionally during the cooking process. When the vegetables are all fork tender, remove the pan from the heat.

3. Serve the sautéed veggies over cooked quinoa, red rice, or pasta, and have your eaters drizzle the sauce over the top.

Teriyaki Tofu Fajitas

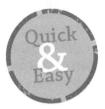

This is a fun twist on a traditional Mexican dish! This recipe is a favorite with the kids. It looks beautiful served with a large green salad. To make this a quick and easy recipe and save prep time for a dinner on a busy weeknight, prepare the marinated tofu ahead of time and store it in an airtight container in the refrigerator. You will need to retain some of the marinade to use for the fajitas recipe; store in an airtight container or glass jar in the refrigerator for up to a week.

SERVES 4 TO 6 ◆ PREP TIME: 1 HOUR TO PREPARE THE TOFU AND 30 MINUTES TO PREPARE THE FAJITAS

1 (12-ounce) package extra-firm tofu, drained

1 cup GF teriyaki sauce (such as Annie Chun's brand)

2 tablespoons coconut oil

1 cup chopped onion

2 cups sliced mushrooms

1 heaping cup sliced roasted red and yellow bell peppers

1 jalapeño pepper, diced (optional)

2–3 tablespoons reserved tofu marinade

Sea salt and fresh cracked pepper to taste

6 GF tortillas (such as Rudi's Fiesta or black rice tortillas)

1–2 avocados, peeled, de-seeded, and sliced

1. Slice the tofu in half, lengthwise, then cut it into eight 1-inch slices. Drain the tofu on paper towels for 5 minutes on each side.

2. Meanwhile, pour the teriyaki sauce into a low dish. After the tofu has drained, add it to the dish and let it sit in the marinade for at least 15 minutes on each side. Use a spoon to pour the marinade over the tofu a few times to be sure it gets absorbed. Retain a bit of marinade for the fajita veggies.

3. Preheat the oven to 325°F. Lay the tofu pieces on a rimmed baking sheet. Bake for about 15 minutes, then turn over the tofu and bake with the over side on top for another 15 minutes. The tofu should be tender and cooked through.

4. When you're ready to make the fajitas, heat the oil in a large skillet over medium heat. When the oil is hot, add the onion and sauté until soft, about 4 minutes. Add in the mushrooms and continue to sauté another 3–4 minutes, or until they release their juices. Add the roasted bell pepper and jalapeño and sauté for another 1 minute.

5. Add the marinated tofu to the vegetable mixture and stir to combine. Add in 2–3 tablespoons of the reserved tofu marinade and let the vegetables simmer for 2–3 minutes to absorb the flavors. Season with salt and pepper to taste.

continues

continued

6. In a small skillet, heat the tortillas over medium until they are warm.

7. To assemble the fajitas, place one tortilla on a plate and fill it with the fajita mixture. Top it with sliced avocado, roll it up, and enjoy!

Sloppy Junes and Beyond

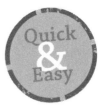

I first tried this recipe out on adults, and they loved it. Then I tried it out on my grandson, and he declared, "Too much spice!" Vegetarian chorizo is spicy on its own, especially my favorite brand, Helen's Kitchen. So if you are making this for the kiddos, you may not want to add the chili powder or cumin. Serve the Sloppy Junes on GF hamburger buns, in lettuce wraps, or over polenta or rice. This recipe makes enough to serve 6–8 people, so if you have leftovers, finish them up by making Sloppy June and Sprout Paninis (page 94).

MAKES ABOUT 5 CUPS • PREP TIME: ABOUT 30 MINUTES

2 tablespoons coconut oil, separated

1 (12-ounce) package vegetarian chorizo, removed from casing

1 cup finely chopped onion

½–¾ cup chopped yellow, red, or green bell pepper

¼ cup drained and chopped sun-dried tomatoes in oil

2 cloves garlic, minced

¼ cup organic corn, fresh or frozen

1 (28-ounce) can diced tomatoes

½ teaspoon sea salt (I prefer Himalayan salt)

1 teaspoon chili powder

⅛ teaspoon ground chipotle pepper (optional)

½ teaspoon cumin

2 teaspoons apple cider vinegar

1. Heat a large skillet over medium-high heat and add 1 tablespoon of the oil.

2. When the oil is hot, put in all of the chorizo and stir it with a wooden spoon for 3–4 minutes. The chorizo has a tendency to stick to the pan and burn, so stir constantly and watch it carefully. Remove it from the skillet and set it aside on a plate. (Note that the chorizo doesn't change much in color or texture as it cooks.)

3. Turn the heat down to medium and add the other tablespoon of oil to the pan. When the oil is hot, add the onion and sauté until soft, about 4–5 minutes. Add the peppers, sun-dried tomatoes, garlic, and corn and continue to cook for another 3 minutes. Add the tomatoes, spices, vinegar, and cooked chorizo. Stir to combine well.

4. Reduce the heat to medium-low and let the mixture simmer to blend the flavors for about 5 minutes. Serve immediately.

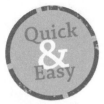

Sloppy June and
Sprout Panini

What is a panini? It's a sandwich! This panini is a great way to use up your leftover Sloppy June filling. You can create fun variations by combining different toppings, but I have offered a delicious combination of toppings in this recipe. For the gluten-free bread, I like to use Rudi's brand; or, try the Hearty Sandwich Bread (page 35).

SERVES 1 • PREP TIME: 5–10 MINUTES

2 pieces GF bread

Sliced avocado

Hummus

¼ cup Sloppy June filling (page 93)

Sprouts

Sliced cheese or vegan cheese (optional)

Coconut oil spray for the grill

1. Lay 1 piece of bread on a cutting board. Place a slice or two of avocado on the bread; you may wish to mash it and spread it on the bread. Top with a small amount of hummus (about 1 tablespoon) and spread it out. Add the Sloppy June filling and spread it out, then add the sprouts and cheese. Place the second piece of bread on top.

2. Lightly spray the top and bottom of a panini machine or indoor electric grill with coconut oil. Put the sandwich in the grill and press it together. The machine should tell you when the panini is done, or grill until the bread is browned and the ingredients are heated. Serve immediately.

Note: This recipe is for one panini sandwich. If you are making sandwiches for more than one person, double or triple the recipe.

Waffle Veggie Panini

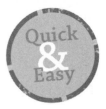

I bought a George Foreman grill years ago, and it somehow ended up at my son Rory's apartment when he went off to college. When he relocated to New York, I was happy to get the grill back! I use the grill often, when the weather does not permit outdoor grilling or when I'm making sandwiches. Gluten-free waffles are a fun, quick, and easy sandwich base. Serve these paninis with a salad of your choice or with veggie chips.

SERVES 1   ◆   PREP TIME: LESS THAN 10 MINUTES

2 slices heirloom tomatoes

2 GF waffles

¼ cup thinly sliced roasted red bell pepper

1 tablespoon capers

1–2 slices fresh mozzarella cheese, 1 tablespoon goat cheese, or dairy-free cheese

3–4 fresh basil leaves

Coconut oil spray for grilling

1. Place the sliced tomato on one of the waffles. Layer and spread out the rest of the sandwich toppings and then put the second waffle on top and press the waffles together.

2. Lightly spray the top and bottom of a panini machine or indoor electric grill with coconut oil. Put the sandwich in the grill and press it together. The machine should tell you when the panini is done, or grill until the waffles and ingredients are heated through, about 3 minutes. Cut the panini in half and serve.

Note: This recipe is for one panini sandwich. If you are making sandwiches for more than one person, double or triple the recipe.

Pizza Three Ways:
Chorizo, Mushroom, and Kale; Italian-Style; and Leek and Mushroom

My goal for this book is to offer you and your family plenty of options, so here are three different recipes for pizza. Feel free to leave off any ingredients that you know your kids will pick off! There are plenty of variations you can do using your family's favorite veggies. You can try replacing a disliked veggie, for example, olives, with something else with an Italian flavor, such as capers. Please note that the recipes for crust and sauce make enough for two pizzas, and each topping recipe makes enough for one pizza. So try out two different pizza topping recipes, or store the extra crust and sauce for lunch tomorrow. The sauce and crust will stay fresh in the refrigerator for a few days.

Hearty Teff Pizza Crust

There are many gluten-free pizza crusts on the market (including Conti's, Rudi's, and Udi's brands), but they all contain egg. If you are a vegan and do not wish to buy a crust, try this recipe. I have made this crust for numerous friends, and they all agree that this recipe is hearty and full of flavor. It takes a bit longer to cook than the store-bought brands because it is so dense—I use teff and sorghum flour rather than potato starch and tapioca—but it is worth the wait!

MAKES TWO LARGE, ROUND 13-INCH CRUSTS ◆ PREP TIME: 25–30 MINUTES

2 teaspoons yeast

1 cup warm water

1 teaspoon organic coconut palm sugar

½ cup teff flour

1½ cups plus 2 tablespoons sorghum flour

2 tablespoons coconut flour

½ teaspoon sea salt

1 teaspoon baking powder

1½ teaspoons guar gum

1 teaspoon chia seeds whisked with 2 tablespoons water (allow 5–6 minutes to gel)

1 tablespoon olive oil

1 teaspoon apple cider vinegar (I prefer Bragg's brand)

Olive oil spray

1. Put the yeast and warm water in a large bowl. Sprinkle the sugar over the top to help activate the yeast. Let the yeast sit for 5–10 minutes.

2. While the yeast is activating, combine the flours, salt, baking powder, and guar gum in a bowl. Set it aside.

3. Add the chia seed mixture, olive oil, and vinegar to the yeast mixture and stir to incorporate fully. Add the dry ingredients to this wet mixture and stir well to combine.

4. With clean hands, gently knead the dough in the bowl and then form it into two balls. Set one ball aside.

5. Lightly spray a round pizza stone or pan with olive oil. Press the dough onto the pizza stone or pan and cover it with a piece of waxed paper. Press your hands against the waxed paper to spread dough out to the edges of the pan. (The waxed paper helps because the dough is sticky. If you don't have any waxed paper, sprinkle a bit of extra sorghum flour over the top of the dough.)

6. When the dough is flattened and evenly spread across the pizza stone or pan, remove the waxed paper. Preheat the oven to 400°F and cook the crust for about 10 minutes. Remove the crust from the oven—it is now par-baked and ready to top! Please note that the crust will go back in the oven for 8–10 minutes after the toppings have been added.

7. Repeat steps 5 and 6 with the other ball of dough, or wrap the dough in plastic wrap and keep it in the refrigerator for up to a week.

Pizza Sauce

MAKES MORE THAN 1 CUP (ENOUGH FOR TWO PIZZAS) • PREP TIME: 25–30 MINUTES

1 (6-ounce) can organic tomato paste

½ can water (3 ounces)

1 teaspoon dried oregano

1 tablespoon chopped fresh parsley

1–2 tablespoons chopped fresh basil
(or 1½ teaspoons dried)

¼ teaspoon sea salt

Fresh cracked pepper to taste

1. Mix all of the ingredients in a large bowl and whisk to fully incorporate. Set the sauce aside for at least 20–30 minutes to allow the flavors to blend.

Chorizo, Mushroom, and Kale Pizza Topping

SERVES 4 • PREP TIME: LESS THAN 30 MINUTES

1 tablespoon olive oil

1 cup chopped yellow or sweet onion

¼ cup chopped sun-dried tomatoes

2 cups sliced mushrooms

½ package (6 ounces) vegetarian chorizo (such as Helen's Kitchen brand)

1 cup chopped kale

1 pizza crust

½ cup pizza sauce

¼ cup Parmesan cheese or Mock Parmesan Cheese (page 201)

1. Heat the oil in a large skillet over medium heat. When the oil is hot, add the onion and sauté for 4 minutes, or until soft. Add the sun-dried tomatoes and mushrooms and continue sautéing for 3–4 minutes, or until the mushrooms begin to soften. Add the chorizo and sauté for another 2–3 minutes. Next add the kale and sauté for another 2 minutes, stirring often. When the kale is slightly wilted, remove the skillet from heat.

2. Have your homemade or store-bought crust and sauce ready. Cover the crust with pizza sauce and spread the pizza filling over the top. Sprinkle with the cheese.

3. Preheat the oven to 400°F. Bake the pizza for 8–10 minutes. Let the pizza cool slightly before serving.

Italian-Style Pizza Topping

SERVES 4 • PREP TIME: LESS THAN 30 MINUTES

1½ tablespoons olive oil

1 cup chopped onion

1 cup diced zucchini

2 tablespoons drained and chopped sun-dried tomatoes in oil

12 Kalamata olives, sliced in half

3 cloves garlic, minced

2 cups chopped arugula

1 pizza crust

½ cup pizza sauce

¼ cup Parmesan cheese or Mock Parmesan Cheese (page 201)

1. Heat the oil in a large skillet over medium heat. When the oil is hot, add the onion and sauté until the onion is soft, about 4 minutes. Add in the zucchini and sun-dried tomatoes and continue to sauté for about 4 minutes. Add the olives, garlic, and arugula and sauté for 2–3 minutes, or until the vegetables are cooked al dente. Remove the pan from the heat.

2. Put the pizza crust on a baking sheet or pizza stone. Spread the pizza sauce over the crust. Arrange the vegetable mixture on top and sprinkle with the Parmesan cheese. It may seem like a lot of veggies to add, but they will cook down in the baking process.

3. Preheat the oven to 400°F. Bake the pizza for 15 minutes, or until it is browned and the cheese is cooked. Please note that if you are using Mock Parmesan Cheese, it will not change in texture when baked.

Leek and Mushroom Pizza Topping

SERVES 4 • PREP TIME: LESS THAN 30 MINUTES

1 tablespoon olive oil

2 leeks, cleaned and diced (about 1¼ cups)

4 cups sliced cremini mushrooms

1 tablespoon chopped sun-dried tomatoes (optional)

3 cloves garlic, minced

1 pizza crust

½ cup pizza sauce

2 tablespoons Mock Parmesan Cheese (page 201)

1. Heat the oil in a large skillet over medium heat. When the oil is hot, add the leeks and sauté for 3 minutes. Add the mushrooms and sun-dried tomatoes and continue sautéing, stirring frequently, for about 3 minutes, or until the veggies are tender. Add the garlic and sauté for another minute. Remove the pan from the heat. Set it aside.

2. Put the pizza crust on a pizza stone or pan and spread out the pizza sauce. Top it with the vegetable topping. Sprinkle the cheese on top.

3. Preheat the oven to 400°F. Bake the pizza for 10 minutes. Let the pizza cool slightly before serving.

Edamame and Vegetable Stew

This hearty stew is great on a cold winter evening. It is packed with protein, and the slight Indian-style flavor is delicious. Serve the stew alone, or put it over quinoa, brown rice, or red rice. I love cilantro, so I add the full half-cup, but you might want to adjust that amount to your liking. Edamame can be purchased fresh or frozen at most grocery stores.

SERVES 6 TO 8 • PREP TIME: ABOUT 1 HOUR

1 (12-ounce) package shelled edamame

1 tablespoon coconut oil

1 cup chopped sweet onion

¾ cup diced carrots

2 cups chopped broccoli

2 cups diced zucchini

1 tablespoon minced garlic

1½ teaspoons turmeric

3 teaspoons cumin

2 teaspoons coriander

2 teaspoons chili powder

2 cups vegetable stock (page 193)

1 (16-ounce) can diced tomatoes

¼–½ cup chopped fresh cilantro

2 tablespoons lime juice, or more to taste

Sea salt and fresh cracked pepper to taste

1. Steam or lightly boil the edamame over high heat for about 4–5 minutes, or until tender. Set them aside.

2. Heat a large saucepan or Dutch oven to medium heat and add the oil. When the oil is hot, add the onions and sauté for about 4 minutes, or until they are soft, stirring frequently. Add the carrots and broccoli and continue to sauté for about 5–6 minutes, or until the broccoli is fork tender. Add the zucchini, garlic, and cooked edamame and continue to sauté for 2–3 minutes, stirring occasionally.

3. Add the spices, vegetable stock, and tomatoes to the vegetable mixture. Turn up the heat and bring the entire mixture to boil. After it begins to boil, reduce the heat to medium-low and let it simmer for 5 minutes to allow the flavors to blend.

4. Add the cilantro and lime juice and continue to simmer for another 1–2 minutes. Season the stew with salt and pepper to taste and serve.

Eggplant Lasagna

Eggplant is one of my favorite vegetables. Grilled eggplant "noodles" form the base for this unusual lasagna! To prepare the eggplant, I use my trusty George Foreman grill, but you can use any grill that's convenient. The Italian flavor of lasagna shines in this dish even though the recipe is a variation on the traditional style. This recipe is vegan, but if you wish to make it vegetarian instead, use cheeses that contain dairy. If you family doesn't eat the entire lasagna in one sitting, any leftovers will store well in an airtight container in your refrigerator for a few days.

MAKES 4–6 SERVINGS • PREP TIME: 1 HOUR

1 large eggplant

Sea salt for sprinkling

3 cups (24 ounces) tomato sauce (homemade or store-bought)

2–3 cloves garlic, minced

2 tablespoons chopped fresh basil

Sea salt and fresh cracked pepper to taste

¼ cup red wine (optional)

1–2 tablespoons olive oil

1 cup chopped yellow onion

⅓ cup drained and chopped sun-dried tomatoes in oil

2 cups chopped kale

5 cups chopped spinach

1 (8-ounce) carton cremini mushrooms, cleaned and sliced

1 small zucchini, sliced

Coconut oil or olive oil spray

2 tablespoons capers (optional)

1 cup grated vegan mozzarella cheese (or dairy mozzarella cheese)

¼ cup Mock Parmesan Cheese (page 201)

1. Peel the eggplant and cut it into about twelve thin strips. Sprinkle each strip lightly with salt. Drain the eggplant on paper towels for about 15 minutes, then turn the pieces over, lightly salt the other sides, and then drain. Rinse well and lay out on paper towels to dry.

2. Heat an indoor electric grill (such as a George Foreman) or outdoor gas grill to 350°F. Grill the eggplant for about 4 minutes on each side, or until it is soft, and then set it aside.

3. In a large bowl, add the tomato sauce, garlic, basil, salt, pepper, and red wine and stir to combine. Set the bowl aside.

4. Heat a large skillet over medium heat and add 1 tablespoon of the olive oil.

5. When the oil is hot, add the onions and sauté them until they are soft, about 4 minutes. Add the sun-dried tomatoes, kale, spinach, mushrooms, and zucchini and continue to sauté until veggies are slightly softened, about 4–5 minutes. Season the veggies with salt and pepper and set them aside.

continues

continued

6. Preheat the oven to 350°F and lightly spray a 9 × 9-inch baking dish with coconut or olive oil. 7. Start layering the casserole, beginning with the eggplant. Cover the bottom of the casserole dish with 4–5 strips of the eggplant. Cover the eggplant with some of the tomato sauce. Layer some of the veggie mixture on top of the sauce, then sprinkle about ½ cup of the mozzarella cheese over the top. Start over with another layer of the eggplant and add subsequent layers until you have reached the top of the casserole dish or run out of ingredients. Reserve a small amount of mozzarella cheese for the end. Sprinkle the reserved mozzarella and the Parmesan cheese on the top of the casserole.

8. Bake uncovered in the oven until the lasagna is heated through and the top is golden-brown and bubbly, about 45 minutes. Please note that you should check the lasagna after 30 minutes because some ovens are hotter than others. If your oven is running hot and your lasagna is browning too quickly, cover it with aluminum foil for the remainder of the cooking time. Remove the lasagna from the oven and serve.

Moussaka

Moussaka is a Greek casserole dish traditionally made with meat, vegetables, and cheese. I developed this version that is modified for the gluten-free vegetarian, but it doesn't miss the flavor! I replaced the traditional meat in this dish with tofu. The moussaka makes great leftovers, and it will last well in the fridge for several days. I highly recommend taking this casserole along to a potluck.

SERVES 4 TO 6   ◆   PREP TIME: 1 HOUR AND 15 MINUTES

1 large eggplant

Sea salt for sprinkling

2 tablespoons olive oil, separated

1 large onion, chopped (about 1½–2 cups)

1 pound firm tofu, cut into small cubes

2 large cloves garlic, chopped

1 (12-ounce) can tomato sauce

1 heaping teaspoon cinnamon

4 egg yolks, beaten

Sea salt and fresh cracked pepper to taste

2 tablespoons butter, ghee, or non-dairy margarine

2 tablespoons arrowroot powder

1 cup soy or coconut milk

2 tablespoons cream cheese or non-dairy cream cheese (optional)

Coconut oil or olive oil spray

¼ cup grated Parmesan cheese or Mock Parmesan Cheese (page 201)

1. Peel the eggplant and cut it into about twelve thin strips. Sprinkle each strip lightly with salt. Drain on paper towels for about 15 minutes. Flip the pieces over, lightly salt the other sides, and then drain. Rinse well and lay out on paper towels to dry.

2. Heat an outdoor or indoor electric grill to medium heat. Grill the eggplant for about 4 minutes on each side, or until it is soft. Set it aside.

3. Heat a large skillet over medium heat and add 1 tablespoon of the olive oil. When the oil is hot, add the onion and sauté it for about 4 minutes, or until it is soft. Add in the tofu and continue to sauté, stirring until the tofu is lightly browned, about 3–4 minutes. Add the garlic and cook for another minute.

4. Add the tomato sauce, cinnamon, and half of the beaten egg yolks to the tofu mixture and stir to blend the flavors. Season the mixture with salt and pepper and remove it from the heat.

5. In a 2-quart saucepan, melt the butter over medium to medium-low heat. Add the arrowroot powder and stir to mix in. The mixture will ball up quickly, so add in the milk slowly, stirring constantly, until the mixture begins to thicken. Reduce the heat so that it doesn't burn. Once the mixture is thick, add the cream cheese and the remaining beaten egg yolks. Remove the pan from the heat and whisk to fully incorporate the ingredients.

continues

continued

6. Preheat the oven to 350°F and lightly spray a
    9 × 9-inch baking dish with coconut or olive oil.

7. Place a layer of the eggplant on the bottom of the dish.
    Add a layer of the tofu mixture and then another layer
    of the eggplant. Use the rest of the tofu mixture as
    the top layer. Pour the thickened sauce over the top of
    the entire casserole. Top it with some fresh cracked
    pepper and the grated cheese.

8. Bake the casserole uncovered for about 35–45
    minutes, or until browned and bubbly. Please note
    that you should check the casserole after 30 minutes
    because some ovens are hotter than others. If your
    oven is running hot and your casserole is browning
    too quickly, cover it with aluminum foil for the
    remainder of the cooking time. Remove the casserole
    from the oven and serve.

Quick and Easy
Kelp Noodle Veggie Dish

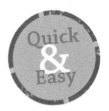

I took this dish to a potluck, and it was very well received! Kelp noodles don't require cooking, so this recipe is quick and easy. Kelp noodles are also healthy to use because they have no fat, cholesterol, protein, or sugar. They yield only one gram of carbohydrate per serving. Kelp noodles provide 1 gram of fiber and up to 15 percent of the daily requirement for calcium, and they contain only 35 milligrams of sodium. Four ounces of kelp noodles provide 4 percent of the daily iron requirement. But not only is this recipe healthy, but it's full of flavor as well! The vegan chorizo is spicy already, so you don't need to add any other spices besides sea salt and fresh cracked pepper.

SERVES 4 • PREP TIME: 15–20 MINUTES

1 tablespoon coconut oil

1 medium sweet onion, chopped (about 1 cup)

½ package (6 ounces) vegetarian chorizo (I prefer Helen's Kitchen brand), removed from casing

3 cups chopped broccoli

2 cups diced zucchini

3 cups organic pasta sauce (homemade or store-bought)

½ package (6 ounces) kelp noodles (about ½ cup), rinsed and cut into bite-size pieces

¼ cup sauerkraut (optional)

Sea salt and fresh cracked pepper to taste

1. Heat a large skillet over medium heat and add the oil. When the oil is hot, add the onion and sauté for about 4 minutes, or until soft, stirring frequently. Add the chorizo and cook for 2–3 minutes. Add the broccoli and continue to sauté for 3–4 minutes, stirring often. If the mixture is sticking to the bottom of the skillet, add either a splash of vegetable stock or water. Add the zucchini and continue to sauté for 1–2 minutes.

2. Reduce the heat to medium-low and cover the skillet so the veggies steam for 4–5 minutes, or until the broccoli is fork tender. Add more water or vegetable stock to avoid sticking, if needed.

3. Remove the cover and add the pasta sauce, noodles, and sauerkraut. Season the mixture with salt and pepper to taste. Continue to cook until the dish is heated through. Serve immediately.

Easy Spaghetti Casserole

This casserole is great with lots of veggies, but if you use a pasta sauce that already has veggies in it, you may not need to add any extra. I recommend using the Slow Cooker Sauce (page 182) for this casserole. I like using Helen's Kitchen Organic Veggie Ground for the protein crumbles because it's organic and GMO-free. Serve this casserole with a green salad for an easy weeknight meal.

SERVES 6 TO 8 • PREP TIME: 45 MINUTES

1 tablespoon coconut oil

1 (12-ounce) package vegetable protein crumbles

4 cups Slow Cooker Sauce (page 182) or 1 (25-ounce) jar organic pasta sauce

4 cups dried pasta (such as GF fusilli)

1 cup Cheddar cheese, Parmesan cheese, or non-dairy cheese (such as Mock Parmesan Cheese, page 201)

1. Heat a non-stick skillet over medium-high heat and add the oil.

2. When the oil is hot, add the protein crumbles and stir frequently for 4–5 minutes. Add the pasta sauce to the skillet and reduce the heat to simmer.

3. Meanwhile, heat a large pot of water over high heat. When the water boils, cook the noodles according to the directions on the package. Cook the pasta to al dente and drain.

4. Add the cooked noodles to the pasta sauce mixture and stir to blend fully. Remove from heat.

5. Pour the mixture into a 9 × 11-inch baking dish. Sprinkle the cheese over the top.

6. Preheat the oven to 350°F. Bake the casserole for 30 minutes, or until the cheese is lightly browned and the casserole is bubbly. Let the casserole cool for 5 minutes before serving.

Simple Pasta with White Bean Sauce

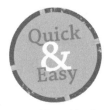

I like to find healthy alternatives to recipes I grew up eating. Creamy pasta sauces like Alfredo and vodka sauce are traditionally made with butter and heavy cream. In this healthier version, white beans are the main ingredient for the sauce, and herbs and spices are added to augment the flavor. To maintain the focus on healthier options, consider using quinoa or whole-grain penne pasta, or spaghetti squash, for this recipe. Spaghetti squash can be made ahead of time and stored in an airtight container in the refrigerator for a few days. When you're ready to use it, just heat it and serve—no additional prep time! If you'd like feel free to tweak the recipe with extra veggies or spices to tantalize your taste buds.

SERVES 4 • PREP TIME: 30 MINUTES

Sauce:

1 tablespoon olive oil

1 cup finely chopped yellow onion

½ cup chopped roasted red bell pepper

¼ cup chopped sun-dried tomatoes

3 cups cooked white beans (such as Great Northern or Cannellini)

½ cup white wine or water

4–5 cloves garlic, minced

¼ cup chopped fresh parsley

½–¾ teaspoon dried, crumbled rosemary

½ teaspoon oregano or tarragon

½ teaspoon sea salt

Lots of fresh cracked pepper to taste

Pasta:

3 cups dry GF pasta (multigrain or quinoa penne) or 1 pre-baked spaghetti squash

½ cup Parmesan cheese or Mock Parmesan Cheese (page 201) (optional)

1. Heat a large skillet over medium heat and add the oil.

2. When the oil is hot, add the onion and sauté for 4 minutes, or until it is soft. Add in the bell pepper and sun-dried tomatoes and continue sautéing for 3–4 minutes, stirring frequently. If mixture is cooking too quickly or beginning to burn, reduce the heat to medium-low and continue sautéing for 1 minute.

3. Add the beans, wine, garlic, and herbs. Reduce the heat and simmer the mixture until flavors blend together, about 5–6 minutes.

4. Cook the pasta according to directions on the package. Drain and rinse the cooked pasta.

5. Pour the sauce mixture into a blender in batches and purée for a few minutes, or until the mixture is smooth. After you have blended all of the batches, return the sauce to the stove and cook until it is heated through. Season with the salt and pepper. Taste the sauce and adjust the seasonings, if desired.

6. Dish into pasta bowls or plates, and sprinkle each serving with a small amount of the Parmesan cheese, if desired.

Roasted Spaghetti Squash, Thai-Style

Spaghetti squash is a snap to prepare and the "noodles" inside take on the flavor of whatever you dress them with. This curry is flavorful but mild, not hot, so even your fussy eaters will enjoy it! For a balanced meal, pair this dish with a protein-rich salad, such as the Edamame and Quinoa Salad (page 72).

SERVES 4 • PREP TIME: 1 HOUR

2 small spaghetti squash (about 6 inches long and 4 inches wide)

Olive oil for brushing

2 tablespoons toasted sesame oil

½ cup finely chopped onion

4 cloves garlic, minced or chopped finely

6 teaspoons grated fresh ginger

½ cup chopped roasted red bell pepper

2 teaspoons coriander

4 teaspoons red curry paste

1 cup organic canned coconut milk

2 tablespoons freshly squeezed lime juice

½ cup chopped fresh cilantro

Sea salt and fresh cracked pepper to taste

Additional chopped fresh cilantro, for garnish

1. Preheat the oven to 350°F and line a baking sheet with parchment paper.

2. Cut the squash in half lengthwise and scoop out the seeds. Brush a small amount of olive oil inside the squash and lay the pieces cut-side down on the prepared baking sheet.

3. Roast the squash in the oven for 40 minutes, or until fork tender. Let the squash rest for a few minutes until they are cool enough to handle.

4. While the squash are cooling, prepare the sauce. Heat a large skillet over medium-high heat and add the toasted sesame oil.

5. When the oil is hot, add the onion and sauté for 2 minutes. Add the garlic, ginger, and bell peppers and sauté for 4 minutes, or until soft. Stir in the coriander, red curry paste, and coconut milk.

6. Reduce the heat to low and add the lime juice, cilantro, fresh cracked pepper, and salt and simmer for 2–3 minutes. Remove the pan from the heat.

7. Use a spoon to scoop out the "noodles" from the squash in long strands and place them in a large bowl. If you wish, retain the squash shells for serving.

8. Pour the sauce over the spaghetti squash noodles and toss to combine. Season the dish with salt and pepper to taste. For a fun presentation, spoon the mixture back into the shells of the squash to serve and garnish with cilantro, if desired.

Spinach and Sun-Dried Tomato Pesto with Spaghetti Squash

Spaghetti squash is a wonderful alternative to gluten-free pastas. The kids love helping to scoop out the "noodles." You can top the spaghetti squash with a variety of sauces and vegetables. The spaghetti squash is richer in nutrients than GF pasta—1 cup of cooked spaghetti squash contains only 42 calories and 10 grams of carbohydrates. It also is high in vitamin A and potassium.

SERVES 4 • PREP TIME: 45–50 MINUTES

1 large spaghetti squash

¼ cup olive oil, plus more for baking the squash

2 tablespoons butter, ghee, or vegan margarine

1–2 tablespoons chopped fresh parsley

¼ cup chopped fresh basil

¼ cup chopped sun-dried tomatoes

2 cups fresh spinach leaves, washed and drained

¼ cup walnuts or pine nuts

½ cup fresh Parmesan cheese or Mock Parmesan Cheese (page 201)

Sea salt and fresh cracked pepper to taste

1. Preheat the oven to 350°F and line a baking sheet with parchment paper.

2. Cut the squash in half lengthwise and scoop out all of the seeds. Brush the inside of the squash with olive oil. Place the squash cut-side down on the prepared baking sheet.

3. Roast the squash in the oven for about 40 minutes, or until fork tender. (The cooking time will depend on the size of the squash.)

4. While the squash is roasting, prepare the pesto. Melt the butter in a small saucepan over medium-low heat. Remove the butter from the heat and pour it into a food processor.

5. Add the parsley, basil, sun-dried tomatoes, spinach, nuts, and cheese, and the salt and pepper to taste. Pulse the mixture until the pesto is blended and smooth. Set it aside.

6. When the squash is cooked, remove it from the oven and let it rest until it's cool enough to handle. Scoop out the "noodles" with a spoon and place a serving of them on a plate. Top the "noodles" with a generous helping of the pesto. Serve immediately.

Roasted Cauliflower and Butternut Squash with Polenta

This recipe not only looks pretty, it tastes delicious. This is an excellent dish for autumn and winter, when the squash is in season. When this dish is served with creamy polenta, it is hearty enough for a main meal; omit the polenta, and you've got a delicious side dish. If you're looking for an alternative to the butternut squash, try delicata squash, as it's mellow flavor will pair well with the cauliflower.

SERVES 4 • PREP TIME: 60–75 MINUTES

1 medium-size head of cauliflower, washed and cut into bite-size pieces (about 4 cups)

1 small butternut squash, peeled and cut into bite-size cubes (about 4 cups)

1 teaspoon crushed or minced garlic

1 medium yellow onion, chopped (about 1 cup)

2 tablespoons coconut oil, melted

1 teaspoon Herbes de Provence

¼–½ teaspoon sea salt

½ teaspoon fresh cracked pepper, or to taste

5 cups water

1 cup coarse cornmeal

1 tablespoon butter or vegan margarine

½ cup Parmesan cheese (optional)

Sea salt and fresh cracked pepper to taste

1. Preheat the oven to 475°F.

2. Place the cauliflower, butternut squash, garlic, and onion in a large bowl and drizzle them with the melted coconut oil. Sprinkle on the Herbes de Provence, salt, and pepper and toss to coat well.

3. Spread the vegetables out on a large baking sheet. Roast them in the oven for 35–40 minutes, or until veggies are tender and browned. Stir the vegetables several times during the roasting time.

4. While the veggies are roasting, prepare the polenta. Heat the water in a 2- or 3-quart saucepan. When it comes to a boil, slowly add in the cornmeal, 1 tablespoon butter, and a pinch of salt, whisking the mixture for a few seconds.

5. Reduce heat to medium-low and cook uncovered for 45 minutes, or until thick and creamy. Stir the polenta occasionally as it's cooking so it doesn't stick to the bottom of the pan. The mixture should bubble once in a while but should not boil over. Remove the pan from the heat and stir in the cheese, if desired.

6. When the squash and cauliflower are done roasting, remove them from the oven. To serve, dish a helping of the polenta onto a plate and put the veggies on top. Season with salt and pepper as desired.

Three Bean Chili

I am a big chili lover, especially in the fall. If you like, modify this recipe by using different beans of your choice, or give it a bit more punch by using half regular chili powder and half chipotle powder. You can also substitute the protein crumbles with tofu or sautéed mushrooms. (Grilled portobello mushrooms are so "meaty" that they make a great substitute for meat alternatives or soy products.) Serve the chili topped with guacamole or fresh salsa. Add some cornbread and a green salad, and you have a complete meal.

SERVES 4 ◆ PREP TIME: 45 MINUTES

1 tablespoon olive oil

1 cup finely chopped yellow onion

1 cup chopped red, yellow, or green bell pepper

2 heaping tablespoons diced green chiles (optional)

1 (12-ounce) package vegetable protein crumbles

1 (15-ounce) can black beans, rinsed and drained (or 2 cups cooked)

1 (15-ounce) can white cannelloni beans, rinsed and drained (or 2 cups cooked)

1 (15-ounce) can pinto beans, rinsed and drained (or 2 cups cooked)

1 (15-ounce) can tomato sauce (about 1 cup)

1 tablespoon chili powder

½ teaspoon cumin

¼ teaspoon cinnamon

1 teaspoon cocoa (optional)

½ teaspoon sea salt

Fresh cracked pepper to taste

1. In a large Dutch oven or stock pot, heat the olive oil over medium-high heat.

2. When the oil is hot, add the onions and sauté for about 4 minutes, or until soft. Add the peppers and chiles and sauté for about 2–3 minutes, or until soft. Add in the vegetable protein crumbles and continue sautéing for 4–5 minutes.

3. Reduce the heat to medium-low and put in the beans, tomato sauce, spices, and cocoa and simmer for 20–30 minutes. Watch your pot as the chili is cooking: it should be simmering not boiling. If the chili is boiling, reduce the heat to low. Season with the ½ teaspoon of sea salt and fresh cracked pepper to taste, if desired. Taste the chili, and when the flavors are blended, serve immediately.

Tofu Chili

I love this chili's robust garlic flavor. If you don't have time to soak and cook the dry beans, use organic canned beans. When using canned beans, reduce the salt in the recipe and rinse the beans well before adding them to the chili. The recipe calls for garnet yams; substitute them for mushrooms if you prefer. I like to serve this chili with avocado and fresh salsa.

SERVES 4 • PREP TIME: ABOUT 40–45 MINUTES

1 tablespoon olive oil

1 cup finely chopped onion

1 cup diced garnet yams (optional)

2 cups sprouted tofu, cubed

1 tablespoon water, if needed for sautéing

¾ cup chopped green, yellow, or red bell peppers

4 cloves garlic, minced (about 1 tablespoon)

3 cups organic tomato sauce

1½ cups organic black beans, cooked

1½ cups organic pinto beans, cooked

2–3 tablespoons diced green chiles

¼ cup chopped fresh cilantro

1 tablespoon chili powder

1 teaspoon dried cumin powder

1 teaspoon sea salt

½ teaspoon fresh cracked pepper

1. In a large Dutch oven or stock pot, heat the olive oil over medium-high heat.

2. When the oil is hot, add the onion and sauté for about 4 minutes, or until it is soft. Add the yam and tofu and sauté for another 4–5 minutes, stirring frequently. If the mixture becomes too dry, add about a tablespoon of water to the pan. Add the bell peppers and garlic and sauté until the yam is fork tender.

3. Add the tomato sauce, beans, green chiles, cilantro, chili powder, cumin, salt, and pepper. Reduce the heat to simmer and cook for about 30 minutes, or until the veggies are cooked through and the flavors have blended.

4. Season with additional salt and fresh cracked pepper, if desired, and serve.

Stuffed Cabbage Rolls

This recipe makes a lot of rolls, so it's the perfect dish to serve at a family function or potluck. These rolls are a bit time-consuming to make, but they are well worth the effort! A couple tips to make the preparation easier: do not overfill the rolls and, when you place a roll in the casserole dish, put the side with the leaf edge down so the roll doesn't fall apart. Cabbage rolls are fun to make—consider involving the kids in preparing this meal. You will all be in for a treat!

MAKES 12 ROLLS (6 SERVINGS) • PREP TIME: ABOUT 1 HOUR AND 15 MINUTES

½ cup tomato sauce

1 tablespoon plus 2 tablespoons red wine

Sea salt and fresh cracked pepper to taste

12 napa cabbage leaves

1 tablespoon coconut oil

1 cup chopped onion

1 large red bell pepper, chopped

¼ cup chopped sun-dried tomatoes

1 cup sliced mushrooms

2 cups chopped spinach

2 cloves garlic, chopped

2 cups cooked rice combination (such as brown, wild, and basmati)

¼–½ teaspoon fresh cracked pepper

½ teaspoon sea salt

½ teaspoon Herbes de Provence

¼ cup Parmesan cheese or Mock Parmesan Cheese (page 201)

Coconut oil or olive oil spray for the baking dish

1. Preheat the oven to 350°F.

2. In a small bowl, stir the tomato sauce and 1 tablespoon of the red wine together. Season lightly with salt and pepper. Set the bowl aside.

3. In a steamer, heat water to a boil and add the cabbage leaves. Steam the cabbage leaves for 5 minutes, or until soft enough to roll up. Remove the pan from the heat and set aside. Be sure the leaves are tender enough to roll up, or they will crack and the filling will fall out.

4. To prepare the filling, heat a large skillet or Dutch oven to medium-high heat and add the oil. When the oil is hot, add the onion and sauté for about 4 minutes, or until they are soft. Add the bell pepper and sun-dried tomatoes and continue to sauté for 2–3 minutes. Add the mushrooms and cook until they begin to release their juices, about 4 minutes. Stir in the spinach and garlic and cook for 3 minutes, or until the spinach is slightly wilted.

5. Add the cooked rice to the vegetable mixture, along with the remaining 2 tablespoons of the red wine and the rest of the seasonings. Stir to combine and sauté for 1–2 minutes. Remove the pan from the heat. Set aside to cool slightly.

continues

continued

6. To assemble the rolls, lay one cabbage leaf out on a cutting board and spoon 2–3 tablespoons of filling on the base of the leaf. Sprinkle a small amount of the cheese on the filling and roll up the leaf carefully, tucking in the ends to ensure no filling slips out. Place the cabbage roll in an 8 × 8-inch baking dish, lightly sprayed with coconut oil or olive oil. Continue to fill and roll the cabbage leaves and set them side-by-side in the baking dish, with the edge of the leaves side down so they don't unroll, until all twelve are done.

7. Drizzle the tomato sauce over the cabbage rolls and sprinkle cheese on top.

8. Bake the rolls in the oven for 30 minutes. Serve immediately.

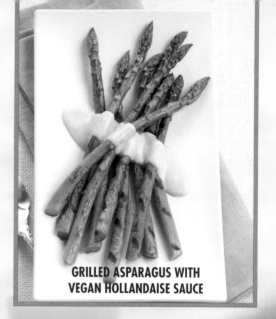

GRILLED ASPARAGUS WITH
VEGAN HOLLANDAISE SAUCE

WARM OR COLD GOLDEN BEET AND APPLE SALAD

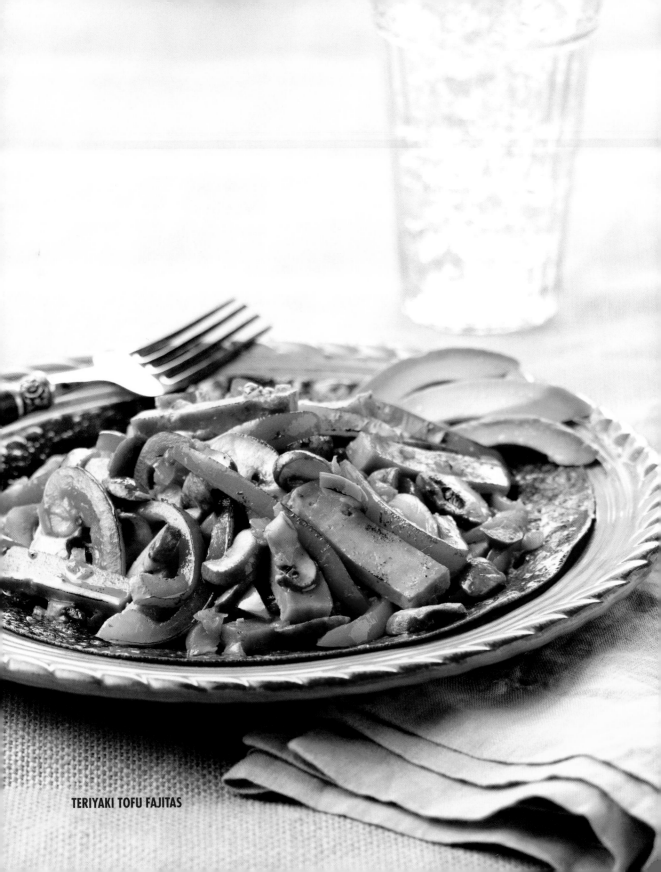

TERIYAKI TOFU FAJITAS

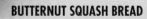

BUTTERNUT SQUASH BREAD

SLOPPY JUNE AND SPROUT PANINI

MU SHU WRAPS, VEGETARIAN-STYLE

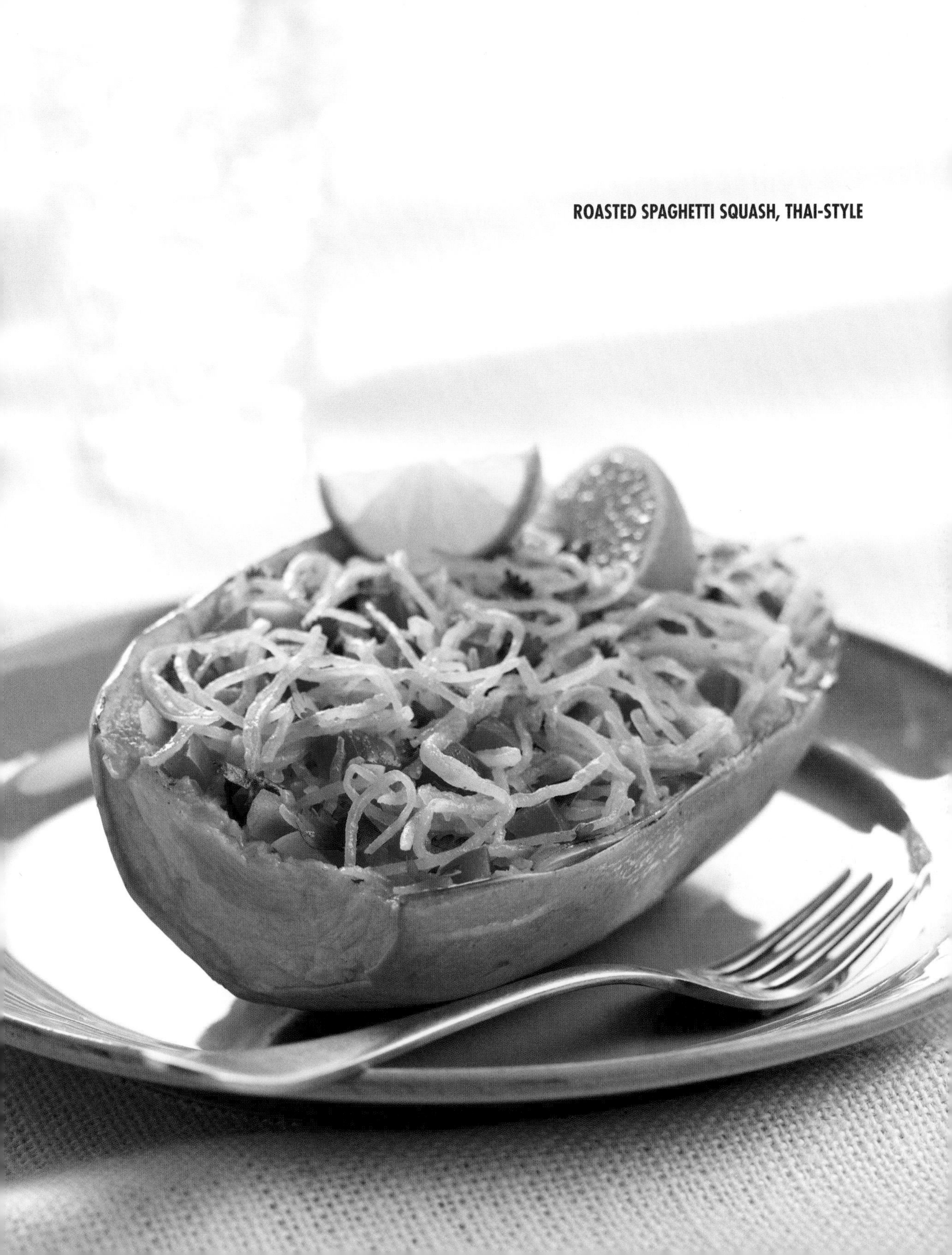

ROASTED SPAGHETTI SQUASH, THAI-STYLE

BAKED VEGGIE-STUFFED PORTOBELLO MUSHROOMS

STRAWBERRY SALAD WITH
MINT DRESSING AND GREENS

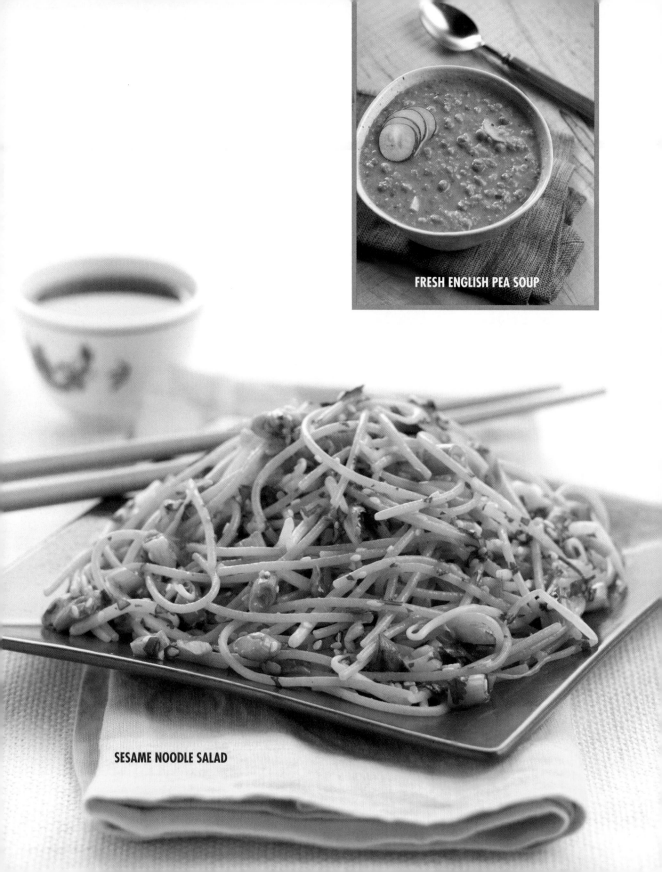

FRESH ENGLISH PEA SOUP

SESAME NOODLE SALAD

Stuffed Green Bell Peppers

The flavor of the vegan chorizo in this recipe is so distinct, I did not add any other flavors except the lime, salt, and pepper. Don't feel you have to use green bell peppers—the filling would look just as stunning in yellow bell peppers. Depending on where you live, this recipe may be best to make in the summertime, when bell peppers are in season. I encourage you to eat only vegetables and fruits that are in season and to buy your produce at local markets.

SERVES 4 • PREP TIME: ABOUT 1 HOUR

4 large green bell peppers

1 tablespoon coconut oil

1 cup finely chopped sweet yellow onion

6 ounces ground vegan chorizo (about ¾ cup)

2 cloves garlic, minced

½ cup chopped fresh cilantro

2 large tomatoes, chopped

2 cups cooked organic black beans

1 cup cooked quinoa

1 tablespoon lime juice

Fresh cracked pepper and sea salt to taste

Coconut oil or olive oil spray for the baking dish

3–4 tablespoons Mock Parmesan Cheese (page 201)

1. Preheat the oven to 350°F. Prepare a 9 × 9-inch baking dish by lightly spraying it with coconut oil or olive oil.

2. To prepare the peppers, carefully cut off their tops. To do this, put a sharp knife about ⅛–¼ inch away from the stem. Gently cut around the stem to loosen the pith and seeds. Pull out the pith and seeds, and discard them.

3. In a steamer, heat water to a boil and set the bell peppers in the steamer, cut-side up so they fit. Steam until the peppers are softened slightly, about 5 minutes. Remove from the heat and set aside.

4. Heat a large skillet over medium-high heat and add the oil. When the oil is hot, add the onion and sauté for about 4–5 minutes, or until soft, stirring frequently. Add the vegan chorizo and stir constantly for 2–3 minutes.

5. Reduce the heat to medium and add the garlic, cilantro, tomatoes, and beans and continue to cook for 3–4 minutes. Add in the cooked quinoa, lime juice, fresh cracked pepper, and salt and turn off the heat.

6. Slice each bell pepper down one side. Open up the pepper and insert some filling. Divide the filling evenly among the peppers. Place the peppers in the prepared baking dish. Sprinkle 1 tablespoon of the cheese on top of each pepper.

7. Bake the stuffed peppers uncovered in the oven for 30 minutes.

Stuffed Zucchini Boats

This delightful recipe is a great way to use fresh veggies out of the garden. Zucchini are in season from summer until late fall, and many gardens run amuck with excess zucchini, so this dish may become a staple in your house! The protein in the veggie crumbles makes this recipe sufficient as a main course, and the boats are delicious served alongside a hearty green salad. You may want to double the recipe so you will have leftovers! The boats store well in an airtight container in the fridge for 2–3 days.

SERVES 4 • PREP TIME: ABOUT 60 MINUTES

4 medium-size zucchinis (each about 6 inches long)

2 tablespoons olive oil, separated

1 cup vegetable protein crumbles

1 small onion, finely chopped

2 cloves garlic, minced

¼ cup chopped roasted red bell pepper

1–2 tablespoons white wine or water

2 tablespoons chopped fresh basil

1 tablespoon chopped fresh parsley (or 1 teaspoon dried parsley)

Salt and fresh cracked pepper to taste

1 tablespoon Parmesan cheese or Mock Parmesan Cheese (page 201)

1. Preheat the oven to 350°F.

2. Cut each zucchini in half lengthwise and scoop the flesh out of each half, being careful not to cut all the way through the skin. Put aside the zucchini shells. Chop the zucchini flesh that you removed and set it aside.

3. Heat a large skillet to medium heat and add 1 tablespoon of the olive oil. When the oil is hot, add the protein crumbles and sauté for 4–5 minutes. Remove the cooked crumbles from the pan and set them aside.

4. Put the remaining tablespoon of olive oil into the pan (make sure the pan isn't too hot so it doesn't splash you). When the oil is hot, add the onion and sauté for 4 minutes, or until the onion is soft. Add the chopped zucchini and continue to sauté for 2–3 minutes. Add in the garlic and red bell pepper and sauté for 1 minute.

5. Add the wine, basil, parsley, and pre-cooked veggie crumbles into the pan with the vegetable mixture. Stir the mixture well, until the ingredients are completely incorporated. Season the mixture with salt and pepper to taste. Remove the pan from the heat.

6. Place the zucchini shells on a baking sheet and carefully fill each shell with the vegetable mixture. Sprinkle a little bit of the cheese over the top of each boat.

7. Bake uncovered in the oven for about 35–40 minutes, or until the boats are soft to the touch. Remove them from the oven and serve immediately.

Summer Veggie Risotto

Risotto is a wonderful way to use a variety of vegetables from the garden or farmers' market. I usually avoid eating white rice because it has low nutritional content, but every once in a while I make an exception for a great recipe! I like to use wine in the risotto because it adds a lovely flavor. If you wish to do that, substitute ¼ cup of the vegetable stock with ¼ cup white or red wine. Most of the alcohol evaporates in the cooking process. This recipe contains only a small amount of protein, so I recommend pairing the risotto with a light bean salad for a more balanced meal.

SERVES 4 TO 6 ◆ PREP TIME: 1 HOUR

2 cups green beans, lightly steamed and cut into bite-size pieces

1 tablespoon coconut oil

1 cup finely chopped onion

1 cup broccoli florets, chopped

1 heaping cup baby carrots, diced

2 cloves garlic, chopped

1 cup diced zucchini

1 cup cubed summer squash

4 cups vegetable stock (or 3¾ cups vegetable stock and ¼ cup white or red wine) (page 193)

¾ cup Arborio rice

¼ cup chopped fresh basil

1 teaspoon tarragon (optional)

2 tablespoons chopped fresh parsley

½ teaspoon Bragg's Organic Sprinkle (or a pinch of thyme, rosemary, and parsley)

Sea salt and fresh cracked pepper to taste

½ cup Parmesan cheese or Mock Parmesan Cheese (page 201) (optional)

1. In a steamer, heat water to a boil and add the green beans. Lightly steam the green beans for 4–5 minutes, or until crisp-tender. Remove the beans from the steamer so they stop cooking and set them aside.

2. In a large skillet or Dutch oven, heat the oil over medium heat. When the oil is hot, add the onion and sauté for about 4 minutes, or until soft. Add the broccoli and carrots and continue to sauté for 4–5 minutes. Add the garlic, zucchini, squash, and steamed green beans and cook for 3–4 minutes. Remove the veggies from the pan and set them aside.

3. Heat a 2-quart saucepan over high heat and add the vegetable stock. Bring it to a boil and then reduce the heat slightly, so it is still hot but not boiling.

4. Heat the large skillet or Dutch oven to medium and add the rice. Stir the rice around the pan to lightly toast it for 1 minute. Add a ladleful of the hot vegetable stock to the rice and stir until the liquid is absorbed by the rice. For the next 30–40 minutes, continue to add one ladleful of stock at a time, stirring constantly until the liquid is absorbed. Repeat until about 95 percent of the stock has been used and absorbed by the rice. Stir the entire time so the rice does not stick on the bottom of the pan and so it cooks evenly.

5. When about 95 percent of the liquid has been used, put the vegetables back into the pan with the rice and add the herbs. Stir this mixture well and allow it to heat through. Add the remaining vegetable stock and keep stirring the mixture until it is fully absorbed.

6. Season the risotto with salt and fresh cracked pepper to taste. Add the cheese, if desired, and stir to incorporate fully. Serve immediately.

Tandoori-Style Tofu with Sesame Tahini Sauce

The word *tandoori* refers to an Indian style of cooking. This recipe for tandoori-style tofu is full of a rich curry flavor and is delicious with the creamy tahini sauce. You can serve this dish over rice, quinoa, millet, or rice noodles. I like to serve this tofu alongside stir-fried veggies and rice—but that's just one of many creative ways to serve this dish!

SERVES 4 ◆ PREP TIME: ABOUT 90 MINUTES, INCLUDING TIME FOR MARINATING

Tandoori-Style Tofu:

2 teaspoons curry powder

¼ teaspoon chili powder

Scant ¼ teaspoon cinnamon

½ teaspoon sea salt

3 tablespoons olive oil

1 lime, juiced

2 tablespoons chopped fresh cilantro

1 teaspoon minced garlic

2 (14-ounce) packages extra-firm tofu

Coconut oil spray for grilling indoors

Sesame Tahini Sauce:

⅓ cup sesame tahini

1½ teaspoons Dijon mustard

5–6 tablespoons hot water

1 tablespoon peanut butter (optional)

¼ teaspoon crushed garlic (optional)

Sea salt to taste

1. In a small bowl, stir together the curry powder, chili powder, cinnamon, and salt to blend. Heat a small skillet over medium-high heat and add these spices. Toast them until you get a hint of the aroma and remove them from the heat.

2. Pour the olive oil into a 9 × 11-inch glass baking dish. Add the lime juice, cilantro, garlic, and toasted spices and whisk to blend the oil with the other ingredients.

3. Slice the tofu into finger-like pieces. The packaged tofu I use is thick, so first I cut the width in half, then slice each half into three sections. I end up with pieces that are about 1 inch wide. To marinate the tofu, either brush the slices with the oil mixture, or put the slices into the dish with the oil mixture and turn them several times, until each side is covered with the mixture. Set the tofu aside for up to an hour to marinate.

4. While the tofu is marinating, prepare the sesame tahini sauce by whisking all the ingredients together in a small bowl.

5. If you are using an indoor electric grill, spray the cooking surfaces lightly with coconut oil, then heat the grill according to directions. If you are using an outdoor barbecue grill, there should be no need to spray it; the oil in the marinade should be enough to keep the tofu from sticking.

6. Once your grill is hot, put on the tofu pieces and cook for 2–4 minutes on each side. Remove the tofu from the heat.

7. Serve the grilled tofu with the sesame tahini sauce on the side.

Spicy Edamame Rice Bowls

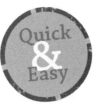

I love to find unique ways to use up leftovers because I hate to waste food! This recipe was developed when I happened to have these particular veggies and leftover rice in the fridge, and it turned out to be a great combination. I used frozen edamame in this recipe, but you can use fresh edamame if you have it. Be sure to buy edamame that is shelled—you probably don't want to take the time to peel off the shells! If you don't have any cooked brown rice on hand, you'll need to add some prep time to cook it, usually about 50 minutes. The combination of lime and cilantro in this dish provide a light and refreshing flavor. This recipe makes rice bowls for two, so double the recipe if you are serving more people.

SERVES 2 ◆ PREP TIME: 25–30 MINUTES

1 cup frozen edamame

1 tablespoon olive oil

½ cup finely chopped yellow onion

1 cup chopped zucchini

½ cup chopped red bell pepper

1 cup chopped kale

½ cup cooked brown rice

1 tablespoon freshly squeezed lime juice

¼ teaspoon red pepper flakes

3 tablespoons chopped fresh cilantro

¼ teaspoon sea salt, or to taste

Fresh cracked pepper to taste

1. In a steamer, heat water to a boil, then remove. Add the frozen edamame to the steamer basket and set them over the hot water for about 5–7 minutes. Remove the edamame from the steamer and set them aside.

2. Heat a skillet to medium-high heat and add the oil. When the oil is hot, add the onion and sauté for about 4 minutes, or until the onions are soft.

3. Add the zucchini, bell pepper, and kale and continue to cook until the kale is slightly wilted and the veggies are al dente, about 4–5 minutes.

4. Add the cooked rice, steamed edamame, lime juice, red pepper flakes, cilantro, salt, and pepper and stir until the ingredients are fully incorporated. Cook over low heat to allow the flavors to blend for a few minutes. Serve hot.

Side Dishes

Spinach and Mushroom Rice Pilaf

The focus of this book is healthy, family-friendly recipes. With that in mind, I developed this rice pilaf recipe, which is great as a hearty side or main dish. I know how challenging it can be to put dinner on the table when you have children underfoot, so this recipe can be made ahead of time and reheated on evenings that are tight on time. If you wish to add protein to this dish, consider putting in ¼ cup lightly toasted pine nuts, or serving the pilaf with a dollop of Cilantro Pesto (page 184). If you don't have the Bragg's seasoning called for, use pinches of thyme, rosemary, and parsley, as well as fresh cracked pepper and sea salt to taste.

SERVES 4 • PREP TIME: 1 HOUR

1 tablespoon olive oil

1 cup finely chopped yellow onion

⅓ cup chopped roasted red bell pepper

1 cup chopped fresh spinach

1 cup chopped cremini mushrooms

1 cup dry wild and brown rice medley

2¼ cups vegetable stock (page 193)

¼ cup red wine (or additional vegetable stock, if you prefer)

½ teaspoon chopped fresh rosemary

1 teaspoon Bragg's Organic Sprinkle

Fresh cracked pepper to taste

1. In a large skillet, heat the oil over medium-high heat.

2. When the oil is hot, add the onion and sauté it for about 4 minutes, or until soft. Add the bell pepper, spinach, and mushrooms and continue to sauté until the mushrooms release their juices, about 4–5 minutes.

3. Add the rice, vegetable stock, and wine to the vegetable mixture and reduce the heat to medium-low. Simmer the rice for about 50 minutes, or until the liquid is absorbed.

4. When the rice is cooked, add the fresh rosemary, Bragg's seasoning, and fresh cracked pepper. Serve immediately.

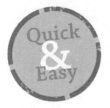

Fall Vegetable Curry over Quinoa

I purposely included several curried vegetable dishes in this cookbook because they use vegetables that are in season at different times of the year. I encourage you to shop and eat foods in season, and I hope you'll give each recipe a try as the vegetables become available. Please remember that my recipes are just starting places—feel free to be creative and substitute with other in-season veggies or family favorites.

   This curry recipe can be served as a side dish or, by serving it with quinoa, made into a substantial, protein-rich main dish. If you use the quinoa, follow the recipe to effectively blend the ingredients together. I like to serve this curry with hummus or dal on the side.

SERVES 4 ◆ PREP TIME: ABOUT 30 MINUTES

1 tablespoon coconut oil

1 large yellow onion, finely chopped (about 1 cup)

3 cups finely chopped purple, green, or napa cabbage

1 cup sliced cremini or portobello mushrooms

1 cup chopped zucchini

2 tablespoons minced fresh ginger

1 large carrot, sliced

2 teaspoons curry powder

1 tablespoon freshly squeezed lemon juice

3 tablespoons organic canned coconut milk

2 tablespoons finely chopped fresh cilantro

Sea salt and fresh cracked pepper to taste

1 cup cooked quinoa (optional)

1. Heat a large skillet over medium-high heat and add the oil.

2. When the oil is hot, add the onion and cabbage and cook for about 5 minutes, or until tender. Add the mushrooms, zucchini, ginger, and carrot and sauté for 2–3 minutes.

3. Reduce the heat to low and add the curry powder, lemon juice, coconut milk, and cilantro and stir to blend the ingredients. Season with the salt and fresh cracked pepper to taste. Let the mixture cook until the flavors blend, about 5–10 minutes.

4. If adding cooked quinoa to the dish, stir it into the curry. Cook for another 5 minutes to heat it through and allow the flavors to blend.

Summertime
Mixed Vegetable Curry

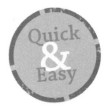

Summertime gives us so many wonderful veggies! I love cauliflower and carrots dug right from the ground. This curry recipe is a wonderful way to blend aromas from the East with veggies straight from the local farmers' market or your own backyard. If your kids don't like mushrooms, use a different veggie, like summer squash or eggplant, instead. This curry is a great side dish, but it can easily be made into a main dish by serving it over quinoa, brown rice, or polenta.

SERVES 4 ◆ PREP TIME: ABOUT 30 MINUTES

1 tablespoon coconut oil

1 large yellow onion, chopped

1 large head cauliflower, cleaned and chopped (about 4 cups)

¼ cup chopped sun-dried tomatoes

½–¾ cup chopped carrots

2 cups stemmed and chopped cremini mushrooms

1 teaspoon thinly sliced fresh ginger

2 tablespoons vegetable stock (page 193)

2–3 cloves garlic, minced

1 teaspoon mellow red miso

¼ teaspoon chili powder

½ teaspoon curry powder

½–1 cup organic canned coconut milk

Sea salt and fresh cracked pepper to taste

2 cups cooked quinoa, brown rice, or polenta (optional)

1. In a large skillet, heat the oil over medium-high heat.

2. When the oil is hot, add the onion and sauté for about 4–5 minutes, or until the onion is soft. Add the cauliflower, sun-dried tomatoes, and carrots and continue to sauté for several minutes, until the cauliflower begins to soften. Add the mushrooms and ginger and continue to cook for another 4–5 minutes.

3. If the mixture begins to stick to the pan, add in the vegetable stock and continue to cook. Add in the garlic and miso and cook for 1 minute.

4. Cook the vegetables until they are all fork tender; this can take 15–20 minutes. Add the chili powder, curry powder, and coconut milk and stir to blend. Season with the salt and fresh cracked pepper to taste. Cook the curry until it is heated through and serve. If using quinoa, rice, or polenta, please cook according to the package directions.

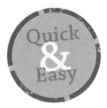

Grilled Vegetable Stack

Nothing says summertime like grilling! This recipe is perfect for the summer because it uses in-season fresh squashes, eggplant, and heirloom tomatoes. Each stack is visually lovely and fun—serve them as an appetizer or side dish at a patio party or enjoy them with your family.

SERVES 4 • PREP TIME: ABOUT 30 MINUTES

1 eggplant, peeled and cut into 1-inch slices

Sea salt for sprinkling

1 medium zucchini, washed and sliced into ¼-inch rounds

1 summer squash, washed and sliced into ¼-inch rounds

1 large beefsteak or Heirloom tomato, washed and sliced into rounds

1 red onion, sliced thinly

¼ cup olive oil

¼ cup balsamic or sherry vinegar

1 teaspoon minced fresh garlic (optional)

¼ cup fresh basil leaves, or more if desired, chopped

1 tablespoon Parmesan cheese or Mock Parmesan Cheese (page 201)

1–2 tablespoons finely chopped fresh parsley

1. Peel the eggplant and cut it into twelve thin strips. Sprinkle each strip lightly with salt. Drain on paper towels for about 15 minutes. Flip the pieces over, lightly salt the other sides, and then drain. Rinse well and lay out on paper towels to dry for a few minutes prior to grilling, to remove any excess moisture.

2. Have your sliced veggies ready. In preparation for the grilling, lightly coat the sliced veggies with a small amount of the olive oil, using a basting brush. Retain the remaining oil to add to the dressing.

3. Heat an outdoor grill or indoor electric grill. Grill all of the vegetables until they are done, about 3–4 minutes on each side, turning only once during the grilling process. Keep an eye on all the veggies while grilling, as some will cook more quickly than others; for example, summer squash and zucchini cook faster than eggplant. When they're done, take them off the grill.

4. In a small bowl, whisk together the remaining oil, vinegar, and garlic. Set aside.

5. You will build four different stacks of vegetables. Begin each stack with round of eggplant, then squash, tomato, and onion. In between each layer, add some of the fresh basil.

6. When all the grilled veggies have been used, drizzle the dressing over the top of each stack. Then sprinkle the cheese on top of each stack and garnish with the parsley. Delicious!

Asian Bok Choy, Mushrooms, and Snow Peas

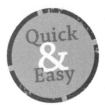

This quick and easy dish will be ready in no time! If you prefer not to use sugar, you can substitute it with brown rice syrup or maple syrup. This recipe includes sake, a Japanese rice "wine." Not all sake is gluten-free. Sake is made from fermented rice, but some companies add barley at the end of the fermenting process to improve the flavor. If you want to use the sake in this recipe or drink some with your meal, be sure to look for GF sake, like Gekkeikan Sake or Rock Sake. Serve this recipe with a rice or noodle dish if you want a complete meal; for example, it's great served with the Sesame Noodle Salad (page 75).

SERVES 4 • PREP TIME: ABOUT 10 MINUTES

8 ounces snow peas (about 3 cups)

8 ounces cremini mushrooms (about 2 cups)

1 tablespoon coconut oil

1 cup chopped bok choy

¼ cup sake (or dry sherry)

2 teaspoons raw or brown sugar

1 tablespoon GF tamari sauce

1 teaspoon toasted sesame oil

½ cup bean sprouts (optional)

1. Prepare the snow peas by removing the strings and cutting them diagonally in half. Clean the mushrooms and slice them in half if they are small, or into ½-inch slices if they are larger.

2. Heat a large skillet over medium-high heat and add the coconut oil.

3. When the oil is hot, add the mushrooms and cook them until their juices release, stirring often, for about 3–4 minutes. Add the snow peas and bok choy and continue to sauté for 1 minute.

4. Stir in the sake, sugar, tamari sauce, and sesame oil and stir to blend. Reduce the heat to medium-low and cook for 2–3 minutes to allow the flavors to blend. Serve immediately, topped with bean sprouts, if you like.

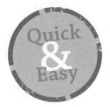

Brussels Sprouts with Maple and Mustard Glaze

Brussels sprouts are chock-full of vitamins—½ cup provides us with 20 essential vitamins, including vitamins C, B, K, and A. Brussels sprouts are also high in fiber, protein, and many minerals. This recipe adds a sweet glaze to the sprouts, so it will be a hit with the kids. I'm sure your whole family will enjoy eating this versatile and healthy vegetable!

SERVES 4 • PREP TIME: LESS THAN 30 MINUTES

1 pound Brussels sprouts

1 cup finely chopped leeks (use the white part only)

1 tablespoon coconut oil

2 cloves garlic, minced

2–4 tablespoons vegetable stock (page 193)

1 tablespoon maple syrup

1 tablespoon Dijon mustard

Sea salt and fresh cracked pepper to taste

1. Wash the Brussels sprouts and peel off the outer leaves. Cut off the stems, and if they are large, cut them in half. (If they are not too big, leave them whole.) Clean the leeks really well. There are often small chunks of dirt found in the folds of leeks.

2. Heat a large skillet over medium heat and add the oil. When the oil is hot, add the leeks and sauté for about 4 minutes, or until they are soft. Add the Brussels sprouts and continue to cook, stirring frequently, for another 5–6 minutes. The leeks and sprouts will begin to brown. If they are browning too quickly or beginning to burn, reduce the heat. Add the garlic and sauté the veggies for another minute.

3. Add the vegetable stock to the vegetable mixture. Reduce the heat to medium-low and cover the skillet. Simmer the veggies for 10–15 minutes, or until the sprouts are fork tender.

4. While the vegetables are simmering, mix the maple syrup and mustard together in a small bowl. When the vegetables are done, add the glaze to the skillet and stir until the glaze covers all the veggies. Cook until the vegetables are heated through. Season with salt and pepper to taste and serve immediately.

Grilled Pesto-Stuffed Portobello Mushrooms

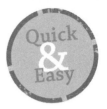

Stuffed mushrooms are easy to prepare and make great appetizers for parties. They also work nicely as a side dish. If you'd like to make this recipe into a complete meal, use two large mushrooms rather than the four medium-size mushrooms called for and serve them with a salad.

SERVES 2 TO 4 (DEPENDING ON THEIR SIZE) • PREP TIME: LESS THAN 30 MINUTES

4 medium-size portobello mushroom caps

½ cup chopped fresh basil

¼ cup chopped fresh parsley

1 cup chopped spinach or arugula

1 tablespoon chopped sun-dried tomatoes

¼ cup Parmesan cheese or Mock Parmesan Cheese (page 201), plus 2 tablespoons for topping

3 tablespoons olive oil

1 clove garlic, minced

¼–½ teaspoon fresh cracked pepper

1. Clean out the "gills" of your portobello mushroom caps to get them ready to grill. Heat your outdoor barbecue, stove-top grill, or indoor electric grill to medium heat.

2. Grill the mushroom caps for 4–5 minutes on each side. (If you're using an electric grill with a small surface, you may need to cook them two at a time.)

3. While the mushrooms are grilling, place the basil, parsley, spinach, tomatoes, cheese, olive oil, garlic, and pepper into a food processor and pulse for 5 seconds at a time, until the pesto is puréed.

4. Heat the oven to broil. Lay the grilled mushroom caps on a baking sheet and fill them with the pesto mixture. Sprinkle the remaining cheese on top and broil in the oven for 2 minutes, or until the cheese is bubbly. Serve immediately.

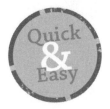

Baked Veggie-Stuffed Portobello Mushrooms

These stuffed mushrooms are delicious and are a great side to accompany a salad or rice dish. If you are using large portobellos, one serving is half of a stuffed mushroom. If you are using smaller portobellos, one serving is one stuffed mushroom. Make sure that you dice the vegetables really well so they fit nicely into the mushroom caps!

SERVES 2 TO 4 • PREP TIME: 20 MINUTES

2 large or 4 small portobello mushrooms

1 tablespoon olive oil

1 cup finely chopped onion

¼ cup finely chopped sun-dried tomatoes

1 cup diced cremini mushrooms

1 cup finely chopped fresh spinach

2–3 cloves garlic, minced

2 heaping tablespoons minced fresh parsley

1 tablespoon chopped fresh basil

½ teaspoon chopped fresh tarragon (optional)

Sea salt and fresh cracked pepper to taste

Parmesan cheese or Mock Parmesan Cheese (page 201) (optional)

1. Preheat the oven to 400°F. Clean out the "gills" of the portobello mushrooms and set them aside.

2. Heat a large skillet over medium heat and add the oil.

3. When the oil is hot, add the onion and sauté it for about 4 minutes, or until soft. Add the sun-dried tomatoes, mushrooms, and spinach and continue to sauté for about 4–5 minutes. Add the garlic and sauté for 1 minute longer.

4. Add the parsley, basil, and tarragon to the vegetable mixture and stir to fully incorporate the ingredients. Season with salt and pepper to taste.

5. Place the mushroom caps on a baking sheet. Use a spoon to carefully fill the mushroom caps with the sautéed veggies. If desired, sprinkle the cheese over the top of the mushrooms.

6. Bake the mushrooms in the oven for 15–18 minutes, or until soft. Remove them from oven and let them cool slightly before serving.

Holiday Butternut Squash with Pomegranate and Quinoa

Vibrant red pomegranate seeds and dried cranberries add to the visual appeal of this festive dish. Roasted butternut squash or acorn squash makes a delicious side dish to accompany the other holiday dishes usually found at wintertime feasts.

SERVES 4 ◆ PREP TIME: ABOUT 45 MINUTES

1 tablespoon coconut oil

1 cup finely chopped onions

1 small butternut squash, peeled, seeded and diced (about 2 cups)

¼ cup chopped sun-dried tomatoes

1 cup sliced mushrooms

1 cup chopped spinach or kale

4 cloves garlic, minced

½ cup chopped raw walnuts

½ cup dried cranberries

¼ cup red wine or water

½ teaspoon dried thyme

1 teaspoon Bragg's Organic Sprinkle

½ teaspoon sea salt

Fresh cracked pepper to taste

2 cups cooked red quinoa

½ cup pomegranate seeds

1. Heat a large Dutch oven or skillet over medium-high heat and add the oil.

2. When the oil is hot, add the onion and sauté for 3–4 minutes, or until soft. Add the butternut squash and sun-dried tomatoes and continue to sauté until squash is nearly fork tender. Add the mushrooms and sauté until they begin to release their juices, about 4–5 minutes.

3. Add the spinach, garlic, walnuts, cranberries, and red wine to the squash mixture, stir well, and continue to sauté for about 3 minutes.

4. Reduce heat to low and add the thyme, Bragg's, salt, and pepper. Stir to blend in the ingredients.

5. Add the quinoa and pomegranate seeds to the mixture. Cover the pan and let the flavors blend for another 3–4 minutes. Adjust seasonings as necessary and serve.

Roasted Butternut Squash
and Brussels Sprouts

This is a fabulous side dish for the holidays. The color of the butternut squash together with the roasted Brussels sprouts is so beautiful. When I made this dish and posted a picture on my GF Facebook page, people begged me for the recipe. It is delicious and oh so easy to make!

SERVES 4 ◆ PREP TIME: ABOUT 1 HOUR

1 medium butternut squash, peeled and cut into bite-size cubes (about 4 cups)

1½–2 pounds Brussels sprouts, cleaned and ends cut

2 tablespoon olive oil

1 tablespoon honey, maple syrup, or brown rice syrup

½ teaspoon fresh cracked pepper

¼ teaspoon sea salt or Himalayan salt

½ teaspoon freshly ground nutmeg

Sea salt or Himalayan salt and fresh cracked pepper to taste

1. Preheat the oven to 350°F and prepare the vegetables. Arrange the vegetables so they cover a 15 × 13-inch baking sheet.

2. In a small bowl, whisk together the olive oil, honey, and seasonings. This mixture is supposed to be quite thick. Drizzle it over the vegetables.

3. Roast the vegetables until done, about 45–50 minutes. Stir the vegetables once or twice with a spatula during the roasting time. When done, the vegetables should be browned and fork tender. Season them with additional salt and pepper to taste and serve.

Roasted Butternut Squash

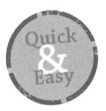

Butternut squash is my favorite fall vegetable. This recipe transforms the squash into an elegant, orange-scented side dish. Squash is a versatile vegetable and can be used in a variety of different ways; use leftover roasted squash in tacos, soups, stews, frittatas, or pasta dishes.

SERVES 4 • PREP TIME: 30 MINUTES

1 tablespoon olive oil, plus more for drizzling

¼ teaspoon freshly ground nutmeg

¼ teaspoon cinnamon

¼ teaspoon sea salt or Himalayan salt

Fresh cracked pepper to taste

1 tablespoon freshly squeezed orange juice

1 medium butternut squash, peeled, seeded, and cut into bite-size cubes

Additional sea salt or Himalayan salt and fresh cracked pepper to taste

1. Preheat the oven to 350°F. Lightly drizzle olive oil on a large baking sheet and set the sheet aside.

2. In a large bowl, add the 1 tablespoon olive oil, nutmeg, cinnamon, salt, pepper, and orange juice and whisk to blend together. Add the cubed squash and toss the squash until it is fully covered.

3. Spread the squash out on the prepared baking sheet and roast in the oven until fork tender, about 20–25 minutes. Stir the mixture a few times during the baking to ensure the squash browns on all sides. Season the squash with salt and fresh cracked pepper to taste and serve.

Stuffed Butternut Squash with Caramelized Onions and Shiitake Mushrooms

Stuffed squash is such a hearty dish. The butternut squash shell is used like a "boat" or bowl that is stuffed with the filling and re-baked in the oven. If your family prefers acorn or delicata squash, no problem—the recipe can be prepared the same way with any winter squash. The best part of this recipe is the filling. What you use for your "boat" is entirely up to you!

SERVES 2 TO 4 • PREP TIME: ABOUT 1 HOUR

1 tablespoon olive oil, plus more for the baking sheet

1 medium-size butternut squash

2 teaspoons coconut oil

1 tablespoon ghee, butter, coconut or olive oil, or vegetable stock

1 cup finely chopped sweet onions

1–2 tablespoons vegetable stock (page 193) or white wine (optional, for deglazing)

1½ cups de-stemmed, cleaned, and chopped shiitake mushrooms (or cremini)

½ teaspoon fresh cracked pepper

¼–½ teaspoon kosher or sea salt

Pinch of fresh thyme, rosemary, or parsley

1 tablespoon Parmesan cheese or Mock Parmesan Cheese (page 201)

1. Preheat the oven to 375°F and lightly coat a baking sheet with olive oil.

2. Cut off both ends of the butternut squash. Use a sharp knife to cut down the middle of the squash lengthwise. Scoop out the seeds from both halves. Place the squash face down on the prepared baking sheet.

3. Bake until the squash is fork tender, about 30 minutes. Check the squash at 20 minutes and every 5 minutes thereafter. Do not overcook the squash because you will be baking it again after the filling is added.

4. When the squash is done, remove it from the heat and let it cool for a few minutes. When it is cool enough to handle, use a spoon to scoop the center of the squash out, being very careful not to cut all the way through the squash shell. Retain the shells and set the set the flesh aside in a bowl. Lower the oven heat to 350°F.

5. Heat a large skillet or Dutch oven to medium heat and add the coconut oil and ghee.

6. When it is hot, add the onions and sauté them slowly for about 15 minutes, stirring frequently. You want to caramelize the onions slowly; if they are browning too quickly before they soften, reduce the heat to medium-low. If the onions begin to stick to the bottom of the pan, add a little vegetable stock or even white wine so they cook slowly and do not burn. When the onions have caramelized, remove them from the skillet and set them aside.

7. Turn the stove up to medium-high heat and add about 1 teaspoon of additional coconut oil or vegetable stock. Put in the mushrooms and stir constantly, until the mushrooms begin to release their juices and become soft, about 3–4 minutes.

8. Reduce the heat to medium again and add the butternut squash flesh that you removed from the shells. Stir the caramelized onions into this mixture. Season with the fresh cracked pepper, salt, and thyme. Remove the pan from the heat.

9. Put the shells on a baking sheet and carefully fill them with the vegetable mixture. Sprinkle the cheese on top. Bake the stuffed squash in the 350°F oven for 20 minutes.

10. Cut each shell in half, so there are four equal pieces, if desired. Serve immediately.

Spaghetti Squash Pasta with Artichoke Hearts and White Wine Sauce

The nice thing about this recipe is that you can do some steps ahead of time in order to speed up the dinner-making process. The spaghetti squash can be prepared and cooked in advance; after the squash is ready, the rest of the recipe is easy and takes less than 30 minutes to prepare. This dish can be altered to add more vegetables or protein if you want to make it a main dish rather than a side dish. For example, add spinach or kale, or add ¼ cup pine nuts or white cannelloni beans to increase the protein.

SERVES 3 TO 4 • PREP TIME: 1 HOUR 30 MINUTES

1 large spaghetti squash (about 3–3½ cups cooked squash)

1 tablespoon olive oil, plus more for brushing the squash

1 cup minced shallots (or onion)

1 cup chopped artichoke hearts in oil, drained

¼ cup chopped sun-dried tomatoes in oil, drained

½ cup white wine or additional vegetable stock

¼ cup vegetable stock (page 193)

1 tablespoon arrowroot powder

¼ cup capers

¼ cup freshly grated Parmesan cheese or Mock Parmesan Cheese (page 201)

½ teaspoon tarragon (or oregano)

¼ cup torn fresh basil leaves

Pinch of red pepper flakes

Sea salt and fresh cracked pepper to taste

1. Preheat the oven to 350°F.

2. Prepare the squash by cutting in half lengthwise and scooping out seeds. Lightly coat the inside and rim of the squash with olive oil. Prick with a fork over the outside of the squash.

3. Place the squash cut-side down on a baking sheet and bake until fork tender, about 45–50 minutes. Turn the squash over halfway through the baking process, if desired. When the squash is done, let it rest until cool enough to handle. Scoop the "noodles" out into a bowl and discard the outer shells.

4. In a large skillet, heat the 1 tablespoon olive oil over medium heat. When the oil is hot, add the shallots and cook for about 4 minutes, or until they are soft, stirring frequently. Add the artichoke hearts and sun-dried tomatoes and continue to sauté, stirring frequently, for another 3–4 minutes.

5. Add the wine and vegetable stock to the skillet and stir to mix. Add the arrowroot powder, stirring continuously as the mixture thickens.

6. When the mixture is thick, reduce the heat to low. Add the capers, cheese, tarragon, basil, and red pepper flakes and stir to incorporate all the ingredients. Season with salt and pepper to taste.

7. Add the squash "noodles" to the mixture and cook until they are heated through. Adjust seasonings as desired and serve.

Sauerkraut Stir-Fry with Kelp Noodles

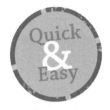

Have we established yet that I love kelp noodles? They are for sale at many different places, including Whole Foods, Mother's Market, food co-ops, Cream of the Crop, Asian markets, and Papaya's—and you can even buy them online from Amazon! You will love that kelp noodles are easy to use and provide a lovely texture. If you can't track them down, substitute them with fresh soy noodles or rice noodles. As you know by now, I am also a big fan of sauerkraut because it's a powerhouse of probiotic enzymes. Cabbage is full of vitamin C and is said to have cancer-fighting properties.

SERVES 3 TO 4   ◆   PREP TIME: 15–20 MINUTES

1 tablespoon coconut oil

¾ cup finely chopped onion

1 cup green beans, cleaned and chopped into bite-size pieces

1 cup sliced mushrooms

1½ cups chopped spinach

½ cup sauerkraut, fresh if possible

1 tablespoon chopped sun-dried tomatoes

2 large cloves garlic, minced

8 ounces kelp noodles (about 1 cup), rinsed and chopped

Sea salt and fresh cracked pepper to taste

1. Heat a large skillet to medium heat and add the oil.

2. When the oil is hot, add the onion and sauté for 4 minutes, or until soft, stirring frequently. Add the green beans and continue to sauté for another 5–6 minutes, stirring often. Add the mushrooms and spinach and continue to cook for 3–4 minutes, or until the mushrooms are juicy and the spinach is slightly wilted.

3. Add the sauerkraut, sun-dried tomatoes, and garlic to the skillet and sauté for 1 minute, stirring frequently.

4. Add the kelp noodles to the skillet and cook until they are heated through. If the green beans are not crisp tender yet, cover the skillet with a lid and let cook the stir-fry over low heat until tender the beans are tender.

5. Season the stir-fry with salt and fresh cracked pepper to taste. Serve immediately.

Basic Slow Cooker Beans

Any time you use dry beans for a recipe, wash and soak them before adding them to a dish. It's important to sort the beans, picking out any discolored beans or pieces of dirt. Then rinse the beans and soak them for at least 6–8 hours. Why? This process helps to reduce the amount of cooking time, and it helps break down the compounds in beans that cause flatulence. Once these slow cooker beans are done, you can eat them as is or use them in a variety of dishes—bean burritos, tostadas, red beans and rice, and more. This is a basic recipe, so feel free to modify it to meet your own needs!

MAKES ABOUT 2 QUARTS OF COOKED BEANS • PREP TIME: 5 MINUTES TO PREP, 8 HOURS TO SOAK, AND 4–8 HOURS TO COOK

2 cups dry pinto beans, sorted and cleaned

1 large yellow or red onion, peeled and diced

¼ teaspoon sea salt

6 cups water for cooking, plus more for soaking

Fresh cracked pepper to taste

Cumin to taste

1. Soak the beans in a large bowl with enough water to fully cover them for up to 8 hours.

2. After soaking, rinse the beans well, at least three or four times, to completely remove the water the beans were soaked in.

3. Add the beans, onion, and salt to the slow cooker and cover with the 6 cups of water. Turn the slow cooker to low and cook overnight, or for at least 8 hours. If you would like the beans done more quickly, cook them on high for 4–6 hours. Season with pepper and cumin to taste.

Seared Green Beans
with Chiles and Garlic

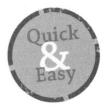

One of my favorite restaurants is East West Café, located in Tacoma, Washington. They serve a green bean dish that I love. This recipe comes as close as I can get to the original—I hope you like the blend of flavors as much as I do. Red curry paste is sold in jars at most supermarkets, but if you can't find it there, try an Asian market or your local health-food store. The dried chiles in this recipe really give it a kick!

SERVES 4 • PREP TIME: ABOUT 25 MINUTES

1 heaping tablespoon coconut oil

4 cups green beans, washed and cut into bite-size pieces

8 ounces cremini mushrooms, de-stemmed, cleaned, and cut in half (about 1 cup)

4–5 cloves garlic, chopped (about 2 tablespoons)

1 teaspoons chopped dried red chiles (or red pepper flakes)

2 teaspoons red curry paste (such as Thai Kitchen)

Sea salt and fresh cracked pepper to taste

1. Heat a large skillet to medium-high heat and add the oil.

2. When the oil is hot, add in the green beans and cook them for about 6 minutes, stirring constantly, until beans are seared and beginning to soften.

3. Add the mushrooms to the skillet and continue to sauté for about 5 minutes, or until mushrooms soften and release their juices. If the mushrooms are cooking too quickly, lower the heat and continue to stir continuously.

4. Add the garlic and chiles to the skillet and sauté for 2 minutes. Add in the red curry paste and stir to fully incorporate it into the mixture.

5. Remove the green beans from the heat and season with salt and pepper, if desired. Serve immediately.

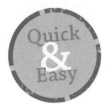

Smashed Yams and Fresh Green Beans

This is a variation of a Croatian recipe my grandmother used to make. She used white potatoes, but the yams in this version offer amazing color and flavor, and the vitamin content is much better too! This recipe is great to serve as a side dish alongside a green salad or casserole.

SERVES 4 • PREP TIME: LESS THAN 20 MINUTES

2–3 medium-size yams, peeled, washed, and cut into bite-size pieces (about 4 cups of cubed yam)

3 cups fresh organic green beans, washed, de-stemmed, and cut into bite-size pieces

2–3 tablespoons olive oil

¾–1 teaspoon fresh cracked pepper

¾–1 teaspoon sea salt or Himalayan salt

1. In a large steamer, heat water to a boil. Put the vegetables in the steamer basket and steam until tender, about 10 minutes.

2. When fork tender, remove the vegetables from the heat and place them in a large bowl. Mash the yams lightly with a fork or potato masher.

3. With a wooden spoon, stir the beans into the mashed yams and then drizzle the olive oil over the top. Sprinkle with fresh cracked pepper and salt and stir to blend well. Serve hot.

Cajun Smashed Sweet Potatoes

This is a fun alternative to mashed potatoes. The seasonings give these sweet potatoes a kick, and the color and flavor will dress up any dinner. Serve them under stir-fried veggies or alongside grilled portobello mushrooms. You could also use this mixture to top a Vegetarian Shepherd's Pie (page 80).

SERVES 4 • PREP TIME: ABOUT 45 MINUTES

2 garnet sweet potatoes, peeled and quartered

4 Yukon gold potatoes, peeled and quartered

½ cup potato water, reserved

1 tablespoon olive oil

1 tablespoon Cajun seasoning

1 teaspoon tarragon

1 teaspoon oregano

Sea salt and fresh cracked pepper to taste

1. Place the peeled, quartered sweet potatoes and potatoes in a large stock pot. Cover them with water and bring them to a full boil. Reduce the heat to medium and cook them for 40 minutes. Drain them over a bowl, retaining ½ cup of the water (discard the rest or use it in a soup).

2. In a large bowl, add the ½ cup reserved water and olive oil to the yams and potatoes and mash them together. When the potatoes are well mashed, add the seasonings and stir to fully incorporate them into the mixture. If you want to spice these mashers up even more, add some red pepper flakes. Serve hot.

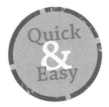

Cauliflower
Mashed "Potatoes"

Cauliflower is an amazing vegetable because it is extremely versatile. I shared this dish with five people and asked them to tell me what the main ingredient was. Only one person guessed it was cauliflower! The secret to making this recipe work is to use your food processor rather than using a blender or a standard potato masher. The cauliflower needs to be puréed to really well to fool your guests!

SERVES 4 • PREP TIME: LESS THAN 30 MINUTES

1 large head cauliflower, washed and cut into quarters (about 4–5 cups)

1 tablespoon olive oil

⅓ cup coconut milk (I like the So Delicious brand)

½ teaspoon garlic powder or 2 cloves roasted garlic

Sea salt and fresh cracked pepper to taste

Dollop of butter or ghee, if desired

1. In a steamer, heat water to a boil. Place the quartered cauliflower in the steamer basket and steam until tender, about 20 minutes.

2. Put the steamed cauliflower into the food processor. Add the olive oil, coconut milk, and garlic and whirl on high until completely blended and smooth and creamy. Season with salt and pepper to taste and add a dollop of butter or ghee, if desired.

Mashed Parsnip Purée

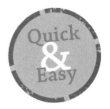

My dear friend Ruth, who taught me so much when I was in my twenties, grew parsnips on her farm, and I learned to love them. Parsnips are naturally low in fat, contain protein (1 gram per half-cup), and are a good source of potassium and fiber. Ruth always prepared them fried in butter, but I prefer the mashed version because they have no added fat. This recipe is seasoned simply, with only fresh cracked pepper and salt; add roasted garlic and rosemary if you'd like more flavor. You can use the purée to thicken soups; just prepare a half-batch if you're making the purée for that purpose.

MAKES ABOUT 3 CUPS   •   PREP TIME: ABOUT 30 MINUTES

6 parsnips

Up to 6 tablespoons milk

Sea salt and fresh cracked pepper to taste

1. Wash and peel the parsnips. Heat water to a boil in a steamer, add the parsnips, and steam them until soft, about 15 minutes.

2. Place the parsnips in a large bowl and use a potato masher to smash them. Add just enough milk to make a purée.

3. Serve this purée as a side dish, seasoned with salt and pepper, or add it to soups as a thickener.

Desserts

Key Lime and Lavender Tart

This Key lime filling is not the bright green color you may be expecting. I don't like to use food coloring, so this filling is the color of the ingredients—but the lime flavor certainly isn't lacking! You can dress up the tart by topping it with thinly sliced limes or, for more color, fresh raspberries and mint leaves. Beautiful!

SERVES 8 • PREP TIME: A LITTLE OVER AN HOUR

1 prepared tart shell (page 150)

1 small package extra-firm tofu (about 7½ ounces)

4 ounces vegan sour cream (about ½ cup; I like Daiya brand)

¼ cup organic coconut palm sugar

2 tablespoons almond meal or almond flour

½ cup freshly squeezed Key lime juice

Pinch of lavender, for garnish (optional)

Mint leaves, for garnish (optional)

1. Have your tart shell prepared and ready. To make the filling, place the tofu, sour cream, sugar, almond meal or almond flour, and Key lime juice in a food processor. Pulse until completely incorporated and the texture is very smooth.

2. Spoon the filling into the cooled tart shell and refrigerate the pie for at least an hour. Garnish the pie with the lavender or mint leaves, if desired.

Tart Shell

Tarts were very popular when I was growing up. My grandmother and auntie made apple tarts and wild blackberry tarts, and I just loved them! This recipe is very simple, and the shell holds up well. You can use it for both sweet and savory fillings. Use this tart shell for the Key Lime and Lavender Tart (page 149) or for a variation of the Strawberry Tofu Parfait (page 168).

MAKES ONE TART SHELL   •   PREP TIME: ABOUT 40 MINUTES

Coconut oil spray for the pan

½ cup organic brown rice flour

½ cup almond meal (page 195)

¼ cup organic coconut palm sugar

5 tablespoons butter, ghee, or vegan margarine

1. Preheat the oven to 350°F. Prepare an 8-inch tart shell (with a removable bottom for an easy transfer) by spraying it with coconut oil.

2. Mix the flour, almond meal, and sugar in a large bowl. Cut the butter into the flour until the mixture resembles small peas. This is easily achieved using clean hands or a pastry cutter. I prefer using my hands so I can feel when the butter is fully incorporated into the flour mixture.

3. Press the dough into the prepared tart pan. Bake for 17–18 minutes and remove from the oven. The tart shell should be browned but not dry.

4. Cool the shell in the pan on a wire rack for 15 minutes, then remove the outer shell by gently lifting the bottom of the pan out of the outer shell. Place back on the wire rack and continue to cool. When the tart shell is cool, add your favorite filling.

Raw Fruit and Nut Cheesecake

Pulsing raw cashews creates the creamy, dreamy filling for this cheesecake. This recipe is easy to make, and the fresh, zesty flavors of lime and orange juice combine to create a sensational dessert! I like to serve this cheesecake with fresh raspberries, but I would also recommend serving it with crushed pineapple or without toppings. The raw crust adds to the earthiness of the recipe without taking away from the freshness of the flavors.

SERVES 8 • PREP TIME: 3 HOURS, INCLUDING TIME TO SOAK THE CASHEWS AND CHILL THE CHEESECAKE

Filling:

3 cups raw cashews

1 ripe avocado

¼ cup coconut oil, melted

¼ cup organic maple syrup

1 lime, juiced

¼ cup freshly squeezed orange juice

1 teaspoon vanilla extract

Zest of lime, for garnish

Raspberries, for garnish (optional)

Mint leaves, for garnish (optional)

Crust:

2 cups raw walnuts

¾ cup pitted Medjool dates (about 9 large dates)

1½ teaspoons cinnamon

1 heaping tablespoon brown rice syrup

¼ cup coconut flakes (optional)

Coconut oil for the pan

1. Place the cashews in a large bowl and cover with water. Soak them for 1–2 hours, then drain.

2. While the cashews are soaking, prepare the crust. Place the walnuts, pitted dates, cinnamon, brown rice syrup, and coconut flakes into the food processor. Whirl until the mixture is completely blended and it sticks together around the sides of the bowl.

3. Lightly grease a pie dish with coconut oil. With clean hands, press the nut mixture into the pie dish evenly.

4. Clean the food processor and reassemble it. Place the soaked cashews in the food processor with the avocado, oil, maple syrup, lime juice, orange juice, and vanilla extract. Whirl until the mixture is very smooth. This may take a few minutes, but keep whirling until the texture is creamy and smooth. Scoop the mixture into a bowl and set it aside. Be sure to scrape down the sides of the food processor so you get all of the cheesecake mixture.

5. Put the filling into the pie crust and sprinkle the top with lime zest. Place the pie in the refrigerator for a few hours. If desired, top the pie with raspberries or mint leaves and serve.

Raw Nut and Date Pie Crust

This raw pie crust is very easy and quick to make. This recipe makes one shell, so it's perfect for a raw pie or cheesecake. You will need to use a food processor to achieve the right consistency for this crust.

MAKES ONE PIE CRUST • PREP TIME: 10 MINUTES

2 cups raw walnuts

½ cup Medjool dates, pitted

1 heaping tablespoon brown rice syrup

1 teaspoon cinnamon

¼ cup coconut flakes (optional)

1. Place all of the ingredients into a food processor and pulse until the nuts are ground and the dates are blended with the nuts. This can take a few minutes. Keep pulsing until the mixture rolls into a ball. Remove the dough from the processor and press the mixture evenly into a 9-inch pie shell. Fill the crust with your favorite filling and serve.

Cinnamon Buckwheat Crèpes with Raspberry Sauce

These are DELICIOUS! I served this recipe to non-GF vegetarians to see if they would notice the crèpes were gluten-free and turn up their noses. Well, that didn't happen—instead, people were trying to resist licking their plates! You can make the crèpes, sauce, and filling up to two days ahead of time and keep them in the fridge until you are ready to use them. To store the crèpes, layer them with waxed paper and place them in a plastic bag.

CRÈPES: MAKES 8 • PREP TIME: ABOUT 10 MINUTES
FILLING: MAKES 1½ CUPS • PREP TIME: ABOUT 5 MINUTES
SAUCE: MAKES 3½ CUPS • PREP TIME: 5–8 MINUTES

Crèpes:

2 eggs, beaten well

1 tablespoon coconut oil, melted

¾ cup regular coconut milk (such as Trader Joe's or So Delicious)

½ teaspoon vanilla extract

5 tablespoons arrowroot powder

2 tablespoons buckwheat flour

1 teaspoon baking powder

Pinch of sea salt

Filling:

1 (8-ounce) container vegan cream cheese

¼ cup honey, brown rice syrup, or organic raw agave syrup

½ teaspoon cinnamon

Raspberry or Blueberry Sauce:

3 cups raspberries or blueberries

¼ cup water

1 tablespoon honey or brown rice syrup (optional)

2 tablespoons arrowroot powder

1. To prepare the crèpes, beat the eggs, and then add the oil, milk, vanilla extract, arrowroot powder, flour, baking powder, and salt. Whisk the ingredients together well; the batter should be thin.

2. Heat an 8-inch non-stick skillet over medium-high heat. Add half of a ladleful of batter (a little less than ¼ cup) into the hot skillet. Swirl the skillet around, so the batter fills the bottom of the skillet and is fairly thin. Cook for about a minute, until bubbles form like they do on pancakes. Carefully flip the crèpe to cook for a minute on the other side. (It shouldn't take more than a minute to cook the crèpe on each side, unless you have used more batter than necessary.)

3. When the crèpe is cooked on both sides and it is lightly browned, slide it off the skillet and cool it on a wire rack.

4. Repeat steps 2 and 3 until the batter is used up. You should be able to make about 8 crèpes.

5. If you are making the crèpes ahead of time, you'll need to store them carefully. After they have cooled, layer waxed paper between each crèpe and store them in a plastic bag in the refrigerator until you are ready to use them.

continues

continued

6. Next make the filling. Whirl the cream cheese, honey, and cinnamon in a food processor until very smooth. Either use the filling right away or store it in the refrigerator until needed.

7. To make the sauce, put the berries, water, and honey in a 2-quart saucepan and heat over medium-high heat until nearly boiling. Add the arrowroot powder and stir well to fully incorporate. Cook until mixture comes to a boil and thickens. Remove the sauce from heat and pour over the top of the crèpes, or store in the refrigerator until ready to use.

8. Once you have prepared all three components of this dish, you are ready to put them all together. Place a crèpe on a serving dish and add a heaping tablespoon of the filling in the center. Fold both ends in and then roll up the crèpe. Place it seam-side down on the plate and serve with a generous helping of berry sauce.

Almond and Oatmeal Cookies, Three Ways

I have created three options for this cookie: jam in the center, chocolate on top, and plain. Bake your favorite one or enjoy them all! Please note that I used a small amount of ghee in this recipe. Ghee is clarified butter that has had the casein and other milk solids removed. If you are vegan, use coconut oil or a melted vegan margarine instead. If you have an allergy to nuts, substitute the almond meal with the same amount of sorghum flour or bean flour.

MAKES 22–24 COOKIES • **PREP TIME: ABOUT 45 MINUTES, INCLUDING BAKING TIME**

1 teaspoon chia seeds

2 tablespoons water

¼ cup ghee, butter, coconut oil, or vegan margarine

¼ cup coconut oil

½ cup brown rice syrup

2 tablespoons maple syrup

1 teaspoon vanilla extract

1 cup brown rice flour

1 cup almond meal

1 teaspoon baking soda

1 teaspoon aluminum-free baking powder

½ teaspoon sea salt

2 cups GF oats

Jam or vegan chocolate chunks

1. Preheat the oven to 325°F and line a cookie sheet with parchment paper.

2. Put the chia seeds and water together in a small bowl and whisk them well. Let this mixture sit for about 5–6 minutes so it can gel.

3. In the meantime, put the ghee and coconut oil in a large mixing bowl and blend together with an electric mixer at medium speed until nice and creamy. Add the brown rice syrup, maple syrup, and vanilla extract and stir until the ingredients are fully incorporated. Add the chia mixture and blend well.

4. Next, add the flour, almond meal, baking soda, baking powder, and salt and mix for 1–2 minutes on high speed to fully incorporate the ingredients together. Stir the oats into the batter with a wooden spoon.

5. Using a rounded tablespoon, drop the dough by tablespoonfuls onto the prepared cookie sheet, spacing the balls 2 inches apart. Press each ball of dough slightly to form a nice round cookie.

6. If you are making the cookies with jam, use the bottom of a rounded tablespoon (or your finger) to form a well in the center of each cookie. Fill each well with a dollop of your favorite all-fruit jam. If you are making the chocolate version of the cookies, lightly press chunks of chocolate across the top of each cookie. Or you can just leave them plain!

7. Bake the cookies for 20–22 minutes. Remove them from the cookie sheet and place them on a wire rack to cool.

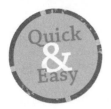

Amazing Flourless Chocolate Chip Cookies

There is no added fat or shortening, eggs, or flour in these cookies. If you are nut-free, replace the walnuts with sunflower seeds. These cookies are wholesome, delicious, and easy to make. Your kids will love helping you bake them—and eating them too! The recipe uses gluten-free oats rather than flour. When you prepare the oats, the goal is to imitate quick oats by pulsing them in your food processor. If you don't have a food processor, you can use a blender, but do the blending in batches rather than trying to pulse all of the oats at once.

MAKES 12 COOKIES • PREP TIME: ABOUT 30 MINUTES

1½ cups GF oats

1 large very ripe banana, mashed (about ½ cup)

⅓ cup sunflower butter (or nut butter)

⅓ cup brown rice syrup

1 cup organic corn flakes (or crispy rice cereal)

2 teaspoons vanilla extract

½ cup vegan chocolate chips

¼ cup chopped raw walnuts

½ teaspoon baking soda

1. Place the oats in a food processor and pulse for 10–12 seconds. Once you have crushed the oats a bit, transfer them to a large mixing bowl.

2. Add the rest of the ingredients and mix well to fully incorporate them. These cookies rely on the brown rice syrup and the oats and corn flakes to hold them together, so it is necessary to refrigerate the dough for at least 2 hours, up to overnight. The longer you leave the dough in the fridge, the better, as the cookies will be more likely to stay together when baked.

3. When cookie dough is fully chilled, preheat the oven to 350°F and prepare a cookie sheet by covering it with parchment paper.

4. Use a ¼ cup measuring cup to scoop the dough out of the bowl. Place each scoop of dough on the cookie sheet, about an inch apart from each other. Press each cookie slightly to make it thick and round. The cookies will not spread as they bake. Place the cookie sheet in the oven and bake for 23–25 minutes. Remove the cookies from the cookie sheet and cool them on a wire rack.

Teff and Oatmeal
Chocolate Chip Cookies

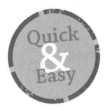

These hardy chocolate chip cookies are delicious. If you do not have oat flour or coconut flour on hand, you can make your own by pulsing GF oats or organic unsweetened coconut in a food processor until fine. It only takes a few seconds, and it's much cheaper than buying flours!

MAKES 12 LARGE OR 24 SMALL COOKIES • PREP TIME: LESS THAN 30 MINUTES

1 teaspoon chia seeds

2 tablespoons water

½ cup peanut butter (or almond, cashew, or sunflower butter)

½ cup coconut oil

½ cup organic maple syrup

½ cup unsweetened applesauce

1½ teaspoons vanilla extract

½ cup teff flour

¼ cup coconut flour

¼ cup GF oat flour

1 cup sorghum flour

2 teaspoons baking powder

¼ teaspoon sea salt

1 teaspoon ground cinnamon

1 cup GF oats

½ cup chopped raw walnuts

1 cup vegan chocolate chips

1. Preheat oven to 350°F and prepare a cookie sheet by lining it with parchment paper.

2. In a small bowl, combine the chia seeds and water and whisk them together well. Set the bowl aside to let the mixture gel for 5–6 minutes.

3. In a large mixing bowl, beat the peanut butter and coconut oil on medium-high with an electric mixer. Add the maple syrup and continue beat, then lower the speed and add the applesauce, chia seed mixture, and vanilla extract and beat to fully incorporate the mixture together, about 1 minute.

4. In a small bowl, combine the flours, baking powder, salt, and cinnamon and stir to mix well. Add the dry ingredients to the wet ingredients and blend well to fully incorporate all the ingredients.

5. Add the oats, nuts, and chocolate chips to the batter and stir together with a wooden spoon.

6. Scoop out a tablespoonful of dough and place it the prepared cookie sheet. Continue to drop spoonfuls of dough onto the cookie sheet, spacing them about 1 inch apart, until the sheet is full. If you are making large cookies, you should be able to fit them all onto one cookie sheet. If you're making smaller cookies, you may have to bake the cookies in two batches. Press each cookie lightly to flatten and round the dough.

7. Bake the cookies for 15–18 minutes. Remove them from the cookie sheet and cool them on wire rack.

Best-Ever Orange Oatmeal Cookies

I took these cookies to my yoga class and everybody loved them. I even shipped some back east to my son, and he begged me for more. Everyone who tastes them wants the recipe—that's a pretty good review! This recipe calls for ghee and egg. If you're dairy-free or vegan, use additional coconut oil or vegan margarine instead. To replace the egg, whisk together 1 teaspoon chia seeds with 2 tablespoons water; let the mixture gel for 5–6 minutes before using.

MAKES ABOUT 18 COOKIES • **PREP TIME: ABOUT 45 MINUTES**

¼ cup ghee

¼ cup coconut oil

½ cup organic coconut palm sugar, brown sugar, or rice syrup

1 egg

¼ cup mashed banana

1 tablespoon fresh squeezed orange juice

1 teaspoon orange zest

1 teaspoon vanilla extract

½ cup almond meal or almond flour

½ cup organic brown rice flour

1 teaspoon aluminum-free baking powder

1 teaspoon baking soda

¼ teaspoon sea salt

½ cup raw walnuts, chopped

¼ cup organic shredded unsweetened coconut

½ cup raisins

1½ cups organic GF oats

1. Preheat the oven to 350°F and line a cookie sheet with parchment paper.

2. In a large mixing bowl, combine the ghee and oil. Add the sugar and blend well for several minutes, until the mixture is light and fluffy. Add the egg and continue to beat. Add the mashed banana, orange juice, orange zest, and vanilla extract and continue to blend the mixture until it is fully incorporated.

3. Add in the flours, baking powder, baking soda, and salt and stir on medium speed to blend well. Add in the nuts, coconut, raisins, and oats and stir together with a wooden spoon to blend well.

4. Drop the dough by tablespoonfuls, spaced 2 inches apart, onto the prepared cookie sheet and flatten out slightly with your clean fingers. Do not flatten the cookies too much, as they are delicious when thick and chewy.

5. Bake for 16–18 minutes, or until golden brown. Remove them from the cookie sheet and cool them on a wire rack.

Apple-Zucchini Bars, Three Ways

I developed three versions of this recipe so it will fit everyone's needs. One version includes eggs and nuts, one is nut-free, and one is both nut- and egg-free. All three recipes are dairy-free. I hope you enjoy the option that's right for you!

MAKES 12 BARS • PREP TIME: ABOUT 15 MINUTES TO PREPARE AND 40–45 MINUTES TO BAKE

Version 1: With Nuts and Eggs

This version produces the lightest bar, but all of the options have great flavor and texture. In this recipe, I used almond meal as the primary flour because it is a low-carbohydrate food and it provides protein (¼ cup of almond meal provides 7 grams of protein).

Coconut oil spray for the baking dish
4 tablespoons organic maple syrup
3 tablespoons coconut oil
2 eggs
1½ cups peeled and grated apple
1 cup grated zucchini
1 cup almond meal (or flour)
½ cup sorghum flour
2 teaspoons cinnamon
1 teaspoon baking soda
1 teaspoon baking powder
¼ teaspoon sea salt
¼ cup finely chopped walnuts

1. Preheat oven to 350°F and grease a 9-inch square baking dish with coconut oil spray.

2. In a large mixing bowl, beat the maple syrup and coconut oil together until smooth on medium-high speed. Add in the eggs and beat to fully incorporate. Add the apple and zucchini and mix well.

3. In a separate medium-size bowl, add the almond meal, sorghum flour, cinnamon, baking soda, baking powder, salt, and walnuts and stir well. Add these dry ingredients to the wet ingredients and reduce the speed to medium-low, stirring to fully incorporate.

4. Pour the batter into the prepared baking dish and bake for 40–45 minutes, or until a sharp knife or toothpick inserted in the center comes out clean. Cool the dish on a wire rack. Cut into bars.

Version 2: Egg-Free

This is the same as the Version 1, but instead of eggs, this recipe uses a chia "egg" and avocado. The chia seed mixture is the egg replacer, and the mashed avocado adds texture and reduces the fat content of the bars. This egg-free version may not take as long to bake, so check the bars when 35 minutes into the baking time. Please note that you can expect the consistency of these egg-free bars to be quite different.

Coconut oil spray for the baking dish

1 teaspoon chia seeds

2 tablespoons water

3 tablespoons mashed avocado

4 tablespoons organic maple syrup

3 tablespoons coconut oil

1½ cups peeled and grated apple

1 cup grated zucchini

1 cup almond meal (or flour)

½ cup sorghum flour

2 teaspoons cinnamon

1 teaspoon baking soda

1 teaspoon baking powder

¼ teaspoon sea salt

¼ cup walnuts, finely chopped

1. Preheat oven to 350°F and grease a 9-inch square baking dish with coconut oil spray.

2. Combine 1 teaspoon chia seeds in a small bowl with 2 tablespoons of water. Whisk together well, then let the mixture sit for 5–6 minutes to gel. It will develop the same consistency as an egg.

3. In a large mixing bowl, combine the chia seed mixture with the mashed avocado. Add the maple syrup and oil and beat together on medium speed to fully incorporate. Add the apple and zucchini and continue to beat on medium to incorporate.

4. In a separate medium-size bowl, stir together the almond meal, sorghum flour, cinnamon, baking soda, baking powder, salt, and walnuts. Add these dry ingredients to the wet ingredients and stir well to fully incorporate.

5. Pour the batter into the prepared baking dish and bake for 35–40 minutes, or until a sharp knife or toothpick inserted in the center comes out clean. Cool the dish on a wire rack and cut into bars.

Version 3: Sans Nuts and Eggs

I used coconut palm sugar in this version to help the bars stay together. Liquid sweeteners like maple syrup cause the bars to be more fragile; the stabilizing effect of the coarse sugar helps to produce better bars.

Coconut oil spray for the baking dish

1 teaspoon chia seeds

2 tablespoons water

3 tablespoons coconut oil

4 tablespoons organic coconut palm sugar

3 tablespoons mashed avocado

1½ cups peeled and grated apple

1 cup grated zucchini

1 cup sorghum flour

2 teaspoons cinnamon

¼ teaspoon sea salt

1 teaspoon baking soda

1 teaspoon aluminum-free baking powder

1. Preheat oven to 350°F and grease a 9-inch square baking dish with coconut oil spray.

2. In a small bowl, whisk together the chia seeds and water. Let the mixture sit for 5–6 minutes to gel and develop an egg-like consistency.

3. In a large mixing bowl, add the coconut oil and sugar. Beat on medium speed until well incorporated. Add the avocado and chia seed mixture and beat well until fully incorporated. Add the grated apple and zucchini and stir on medium speed for 1–2 minutes to blend the ingredients together.

4. In a separate medium-size bowl, combine the flour, cinnamon, salt, baking soda, and baking powder. Add these dry ingredients to the wet ingredients and blend the mixture well to fully incorporate all the ingredients.

5. Pour the batter into the prepared baking dish and spread it out evenly. Bake for 30–35 minutes, or until a sharp knife or toothpick in the center comes out clean. Cool the baking dish on a wire rack and cut into bars.

Pumpkin Bars

My grandson is a bit of a picky eater, but he can't get enough of these bars! He liked them so much that I had to send half the batch home with him so he could enjoy them for several days. These bars store well in an airtight container at room temperature. If you want, you can serve this as a pumpkin cake rather than cutting it into bars; top it with cashew cream or a light glaze of your choosing.

MAKES 24 BARS • PREP TIME: 35 MINUTES

Coconut oil spray for the baking dish

¼ cup vegan buttery spread, ghee, or butter

⅓–½ cup organic maple syrup (depending on your sweet tooth)

¼ cup mashed ripe banana

2 eggs (or 2 teaspoons chia seeds whisked with 4 tablespoons water; allow 5–6 minutes to gel)

1½ cups organic cooked pumpkin

1 teaspoon vanilla extract

⅓ cup coconut flour

1 cup sorghum flour

⅓ cup almond meal

1 tablespoon golden flax seeds

1 teaspoon xanthum gum

1 teaspoon baking soda

2 teaspoons baking powder

2 teaspoons cinnamon

¼ teaspoon ground ginger

¼ teaspoon nutmeg

¼ teaspoon sea salt

½ cup coconut milk (or soy, hemp, or dairy milk)

1. Preheat the oven to 350°F and lightly spray a 9-inch square baking dish with coconut oil.

2. Place the buttery spread in a large mixing bowl along with the maple syrup. Using an electric mixer, blend on high speed until the ingredients are light and fluffy. Add the mashed banana and egg (or egg substitute) and continue to beat until fully incorporated. Add the pumpkin and vanilla extract and mix well to blend.

3. In a smaller bowl, combine the flours, almond meal, flax seeds, xanthum gum, baking soda, baking powder, cinnamon, ginger, nutmeg, and salt. Stir to mix well.

4. Slowly add some of the milk and some of the dry ingredients to the liquid ingredients. Alternate adding milk and dry ingredients, and beat to mix after each addition. Beat well to fully incorporate all the ingredients.

5. Pour the batter into the prepared baking dish and bake for about 25 minutes, or until a toothpick or sharp knife inserted in the center comes out clean. Cool the baking dish on a wire rack and cut into bars.

Chocolate
Puffed Rice Treats

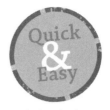

This recipe, with all the appeal of marshmallow rice treats, will be loved by your kids! The basic recipe is a good starting point, but keep in mind that there are so many different variations you can make, such as adding pumpkin seeds, walnuts, sesame seeds, or raisins. If you have an allergy to nuts, try using sunflower seed or sesame seed butter instead—they are both delicious!

MAKES 16–20 SQUARES • PREP TIME: 10 MINUTES, PLUS COOLING TIME

Coconut oil spray for the pan

½ cup vegan chocolate chips (such as Enjoy Life Foods brand)

¼ cup brown rice syrup

¼ cup organic maple syrup

½ cup nut or seed butter (peanut, cashew, almond, sesame seed, or sunflower seed)

3 cups puffed rice cereal (unsweetened)

1. Lightly spray a 9-inch square pan with coconut oil.

2. Heat a 2-quart saucepan over medium-low heat and add the chocolate chips, rice syrup, maple syrup, and nut butter. Stir until mixture melts together, about 4–5 minutes. Be careful not to scorch the mixture. Remove the saucepan from the heat.

3. Stir in the puffed rice, making sure the melted mixture coats it well. Pour the puffed rice mixture into the prepared pan and spread it out evenly and press it down. Let it cool completely, then cut it into squares.

Coconut Macaroons

This easy recipe can be eaten raw or baked, so take your pick! Some of my taste-testers preferred the baked version and others the raw, so in the end, it was a draw! If you are trying to cut down on sweets, reduce the brown rice syrup in this recipe by ¼ cup.

MAKES TWO DOZEN COOKIES ◆ **PREP TIME: 30 MINUTES FOR BAKED; 15 MINUTES FOR RAW**

3 cups organic shredded unsweetened coconut

1½ cups almond meal (page 195)

1 cup brown rice syrup

2 teaspoons vanilla extract

½ teaspoon sea salt

1 teaspoon baking soda

1. Put all of the ingredients into a large mixing bowl and stir together well, until the ingredients are completely incorporated. Wash your hands; you will need to form the mixture into balls, and it is very sticky.

2. For the raw macaroons: Spoon a small amount (about 2 teaspoons) into your hands and roll it into a ball. Place the ball on a platter and continue to roll the mixture into balls until you have used it all. Serve, or store the macaroons in an airtight container. No need to refrigerate them because they contain no fat or eggs.

3. For the baked coconut macaroons: Preheat oven to 350°F and line a cookie sheet with parchment paper.

4. Spoon a tablespoon of the coconut mixture and place it on the cookie sheet. Press it slightly to flatten it and make it round. Repeat until you have used all the dough (you may need to bake them in batches). Leave a space of 1½ inches between the cookies, as they will flatten out while they bake.

5. Bake the macaroons for 13–15 minutes. Cool completely on the parchment paper. If you try to remove the cookies from the parchment paper before they cool, they will stick. Store the macaroons in an airtight container at room temperature.

Creamy Quinoa Pudding

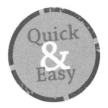

This pudding is technically a dessert, but I must confess that I also like it for breakfast! It's chock-full of protein because the main ingredient is quinoa. With the addition of a few raspberries or blueberries, this pudding makes for a lovely quick meal in the morning. If you do not want to include the egg, replace it with 1 teaspoon chia seeds whisked together with 2 tablespoons water; set the mixture aside for 5–6 minutes to allow it to gel before using.

SERVES 6 TO 8 • PREP TIME: 30 MINUTES, PLUS 3 HOURS IN FRIDGE (OPTIONAL)

¾ cup quinoa (red or white)

1 (13.5-ounce) can coconut milk

2 cups non-dairy coconut milk or whole milk

¼ cup organic coconut palm sugar or maple syrup

1 egg, beaten (optional)

½ teaspoon cinnamon, or more to taste

¼ teaspoon cardamom

1 tablespoon arrowroot powder

½ cup finely chopped pitted Medjool dates

Cinnamon, for garnish (optional)

1. Rinse the quinoa well in a strainer, then add it to a 2-quart saucepan. Put in the canned coconut milk and 1½ cups of the non-dairy coconut milk and stir.

2. Heat the saucepan over medium heat until mixture comes to a boil. Reduce the heat to medium-low and simmer for 15 minutes.

3. While the quinoa is cooking, stir together the remaining half-cup of non-dairy coconut milk, sugar, egg, cinnamon, cardamom, and arrowroot powder. Whisk together well.

4. After the quinoa has cooked 15 minutes, reduce the heat to low. While stirring constantly, add in the milk and sugar mixture. Continue to cook and stir for about 5 minutes, or until the mixture simmers and begins to thicken. Remove the mixture from the heat and add in the dates.

5. Pour the pudding into a medium-size bowl and set aside to cool. If you are serving the pudding warm, allow it to cool for 10 minutes before serving. If you are planning to serve the pudding cold (my preference), cover the pudding with waxed paper and refrigerate it for at least 2–3 hours. When ready to serve, sprinkle with additional cinnamon, if desired.

Delicious Dairy-Free Chocolate Pudding

I worked hard to come up with a pudding that tastes so good you don't know it's good for you! I also wanted to be sure that it was easy to make and that its great taste and smooth texture would pass the inspection of the kiddos in the family. I think I've got a winner with this recipe!

**SERVES 4 • PREP TIME: ABOUT 10 MINUTES TO PREPARE,
PLUS 2–3 HOURS TO SET UP IN THE FRIDGE**

¾ cup vegan chocolate chips

10 ounces sprouted extra-firm tofu

¼ cup honey, brown rice syrup, or maple syrup

½ teaspoon vanilla extract

½ cup dairy-free sour cream

¾ teaspoon cinnamon

Dash of chili powder

1 tablespoon peanut butter or tahini (optional)

Fresh mint leaves, for garnish (optional)

1. Melt the chocolate chips in a double boiler and set aside.

2. Slice the tofu and drain it on paper towels to absorb the liquid for about 5 minutes. Press the tofu to express any remaining fluid.

3. Transfer the tofu to a food processor and whirl it until smooth. Add the honey, vanilla extract, and sour cream and whirl for a minute to blend the ingredients together well. Add the melted chocolate, cinnamon, chili powder, and peanut butter and whirl until the mixture is completely smooth.

4. Spoon the pudding into small bowls and place them in the refrigerator to cool for 2–3 hours. Garnish with fresh mint leaves, if desired.

Strawberry Coconut Pudding

Need a treat for the kids or a dessert for a dinner party? This recipe is easy to make and looks wonderful presented in cocktail glasses! This recipe only makes four servings, so if you want to serve more, double the recipe.

SERVES 4 ◆ **PREP TIME: ABOUT 15 MINUTES TO PREPARE, PLUS 1 HOUR TO CHILL**

½ cup coconut cream

¼ cup vegan sour cream or Greek yogurt (plain)

½ cup organic frozen orange juice concentrate

2 cups fresh strawberries, cleaned and sliced in half (reserve a few slices for the garnish)

2 tablespoons arrowroot powder

¼ teaspoon vanilla extract

Fresh mint leaves, for garnish (optional)

1. Put all of the ingredients except the arrowroot powder and vanilla extract into a food processor and purée until smooth (reserve a few strawberries to slice for a garnish).

2. Pour the mixture into a 2-quart saucepan and heat over medium heat, until nearly boiling.

3. Add the arrowroot powder to the saucepan and slowly whisk to fully incorporate. Bring the mixture to a boil, stirring constantly. When the mixture is thick, remove it from the heat.

4. Add the vanilla extract and mix to blend in.

5. Allow the pudding to cool slightly before pouring it into four ramekins or other small serving dishes. Cover the top of the pudding with waxed paper so a film doesn't form on top and refrigerate the pudding until chilled, about an hour. Garnish with fresh mint leaves or sliced strawberries, if desired.

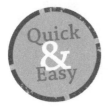

Strawberry Tofu Parfait

This parfait is super quick and easy to make. I recommend using strawberries in this recipe, but I have also made it with a mix of pomegranate seeds, strawberries, and blueberries. If you want to make a tart, you can put this filling into the tart shell found on page 150. If you do make a tart, omit the pineapple; layer the mango on the bottom of the tart shell, then put the filling on top. Delicious!

SERVES 4 • PREP TIME: 15 MINUTES

16 ounces extra-firm tofu, drained

¼ cup organic coconut palm sugar

2 cups fresh strawberries, cleaned and sliced in half (reserve ¼ cup for top)

¼ cup cream cheese (vegan or dairy)

1 teaspoon vanilla extract

½ teaspoon cinnamon

1 mango, peeled and sliced

2 cups chunked pineapple

Fresh mint leaves, for garnish (optional)

1. Put the tofu, sugar, strawberries, cream cheese, vanilla extract, and cinnamon into a food processor and whirl until mixture is fully incorporated and smooth, about 1–2 minutes.

2. Pour a small amount of the mixture into either parfait glasses or a nice glass bowl. Top the mixture with a layer of mango, then more parfait, then a layer of pineapple. Finish with a layer of the parfait. Add the sliced strawberries to the top. Garnish with fresh mint, if desired.

Tropical Banana and Mango Pudding

This pudding is made with tofu instead of the traditional milk and tapioca, so the recipe contains less starch and more complex carbohydrates. When you add the vegan cream cheese in this recipe, start with two tablespoons and taste; if you like a creamier pudding, add more. This recipe will be a hit with your kids and makes a wholesome afternoon snack.

MAKES 3 CUPS (SERVES 4 TO 5) ◆ **PREP TIME: ABOUT 5 MINUTES TO PREPARE AND UP TO 1 HOUR TO CHILL**

1 very ripe mango

1 (14-ounce) package organic medium-firm tofu, crumbled

4 tablespoons freshly squeezed lime juice

¼ cup organic coconut palm sugar

2–3 tablespoons vegan cream cheese

½ teaspoon vanilla extract

1 very ripe banana

Pinch of cardamom or cinnamon

Lime zest or fresh blueberries, for garnish (optional)

1. Pit and peel the mango and put it into a food processor. Pulse until smooth.

2. Add the rest of the ingredients to the food processor (except for the garnish) and whirl quickly until the mixture is well-blended and very smooth.

3. Pour the pudding into individual serving dishes and refrigerate them for about 1 hour, or until chilled. Top with lime zest or fresh blueberries, if desired, and serve.

Snacks, Sauces, Pantry Staples, and Everything Else

White Bean Dip

Serve this dip with carrots, celery, apple slices, or rice crackers for a great after-school snack. Rice crackers are not complex carbs, so I recommend veggies; but if your active kids need a boost of energy, crackers will certainly do the trick! If you don't have cooked white beans in the house, you can use organic canned beans.

MAKES 3 CUPS • PREP TIME: LESS THAN 5 MINUTES

1½ cups cooked organic white kidney beans (or 1 [15-ounce] can white kidney beans, drained and rinsed)

1½ cups cooked organic garbanzo beans (or 1 [15-ounce] can garbanzo beans, drained and rinsed)

¼ cup sesame tahini or sunflower seed butter (page 197)

½ cup freshly squeezed lime juice

1–2 tablespoons olive oil

1 teaspoon minced garlic (from 2–3 cloves of fresh garlic)

½ teaspoon sea salt

1½ teaspoons hot or spicy paprika

2 teaspoons cumin

3–4 tablespoons tamari sauce

1. Place all of the ingredients in a food processor and pulse until completely smooth. Store in an airtight container in the refrigerator until ready to serve.

Spicy Black Bean Dip

If you are making this recipe to take to a party and you are using dried beans, make sure you start the day before to allow for soaking and cooking time. If using organic canned black beans, this recipe can be made in less than 5 minutes, but omit the additional salt. If you want more of a kick in your dip, add hot sauce.

MAKES A LITTLE OVER 3 CUPS • PREP TIME: 5 MINUTES

3 cups cooked organic black beans (or 2 [15-ounce] cans black beans, drained and rinsed)

3 cloves garlic, minced

½ cup chopped fresh cilantro

2 tablespoons freshly squeezed lime juice

1 teaspoon ground cumin

1–2 teaspoons red chili pepper flakes

¼ teaspoon ground cinnamon

¼ teaspoon sea salt

Fresh cracked pepper to taste

1. Pulse all of the ingredients together in a food processor until smooth and creamy. Season with salt and pepper to taste. Serve this dip with veggies or chips.

Sun-Dried Tomato Hummus

This recipe is easy and takes about 5 minutes to prepare, so you can whip it up for an impromptu appetizer or a healthy snack for your kids. This dip is great served with carrot sticks and apple slices, or spread onto celery. If you use canned beans, please reduce or omit the additional salt called for in the recipe.

MAKES ABOUT 2½ CUPS   •   PREP TIME: 5 MINUTES

2 cups cooked garbanzo beans (or 2 [15-ounce] cans garbanzo beans, drained and rinsed)

¼ cup sesame tahini

¼ cup oil-packed sun-dried tomatoes, drained

2 tablespoons chopped fresh basil leaves

¼ cup freshly squeezed lemon juice

2 cloves garlic

1–2 tablespoons olive oil

¼ teaspoon sea salt

Fresh cracked pepper to taste

Warm water (optional)

1. Place all of the ingredients in a food processor (except the water) and pulse until very smooth and creamy. If the hummus is too thick, thin it slightly by adding a bit more olive oil or a small amount of warm water. Season with salt and fresh cracked pepper to taste and serve.

Marinated Heirloom Tomatoes

Summer is the best time for tomatoes. I love heirloom tomatoes on just about everything—from sandwiches to salads to pizza! Serve these tomatoes on top of fresh organic arugula or other in-season greens. I don't like to use a lot of dressing; if the amount of dressing in the recipe isn't enough for you, double the amounts of the oil and vinegar. You can always save it for later if you make too much. For a dairy-free version, sprinkle Mock Parmesan Cheese (page 201) or another non-dairy cheese on top.

SERVES 4   •   PREP TIME: 1 HOUR 5 MINUTES

5–6 large heirloom tomatoes

½–⅔ cup chopped or torn fresh basil

2 tablespoons capers

2–3 cloves garlic, minced

⅛ cup organic olive oil

⅛ cup balsamic vinegar

½ cup feta, Parmesan cheese, or non-dairy cheese substitute

Fresh cracked pepper and sea salt to taste

1. Slice the tomatoes into rounds and place them in a bowl. Add the basil, capers, and garlic.

2. Put the olive oil and balsamic vinegar into a small bowl (or jar) and whisk well (or shake vigorously) to fully incorporate the two together.

3. Pour the mixture over the tomatoes and place the bowl in the refrigerator to marinate. Marinate for at least an hour.

4. Place some greens on a plate or serving dish and then add the tomato mixture. Sprinkle the cheese over the top and season with fresh cracked pepper and salt to taste.

Beet Chips

My favorite beets to use for beet chips are golden beets, but red beets make delicious chips too—and a combo of both kinds is especially nice. Send these chips to school with your kids or serve them as an appetizer at your next family gathering. These beet chips are much more nutritious than potato chips.

SERVES 3 TO 4 • PREP TIME: ABOUT 40 MINUTES

5–6 beets, washed, peeled, and thinly sliced (about 4 cups)

2–3 teaspoons organic coconut oil, melted

¼–½ teaspoon sea salt

Lots of fresh cracked pepper to taste

1. Preheat oven to 400°F.

2. Put the sliced beets in a large bowl and drizzle them with the oil. Sprinkle them with salt and pepper. Toss the beets to coat.

3. Arrange the beets on a baking sheet. Bake them about 15 minutes, use a spatula to flip over the chips, and bake for another 15–20 minutes, or until the chips are crispy.

4. Keep a close eye on the chips during the baking time. If some of the chips bake more quickly than others, remove those from the oven and place them on a paper towel. We don't want them burning while the others finish cooking! When all of the chips are crispy, remove them from the baking sheet and drain them on a paper towel. Enjoy!

Parmesan Kale Chips

I can't guarantee these kale chips will be your kids' favorite snack—but if they like kale, they will love this recipe! I used Mock Parmesan Cheese (page 201) in this recipe, but you can use regular Parmesan if you'd like.

MAKES ABOUT 3 CUPS • PREP TIME: ABOUT 30 MINUTES

1 bunch kale, washed and chopped into bite-size pieces (6–8 cups)

1 tablespoon extra virgin olive oil

¼ cup Mock Parmesan Cheese (page 201)

Fresh cracked pepper to taste

1. Preheat oven to 350°F and line a cookie sheet with parchment paper.

2. Place the washed, chopped kale in a large bowl. Drizzle the olive oil over the top and sprinkle with the cheese and fresh cracked pepper. Toss to combine.

3. Arrange the pieces of kale in an even layer on the prepared cookie sheet. Bake for 20–25 minutes, or until crunchy. Stir every few minutes to ensure the kale chips bake evenly. Chips should be crisp but not burned. Let the chips cool before serving.

Anti-Inflammatory Green Smoothie

Parsley and cinnamon both have a lot of anti-inflammatory properties. This smoothie can easily be adapted to suit your tastes by adding other berries, using other green leafy vegetables, or adding flax seeds instead of chia seeds. You can turn it into a green protein drink by adding your favorite GF vegetarian or vegan protein powder. Be creative and think green!

MAKES FOUR 8-OUNCE SERVINGS ◆ PREP TIME: 5 MINUTES

2½ cups water

1 cup chopped kale

½ cup parsley

1 teaspoon chia seeds

1 cup frozen blueberries

1 banana (optional)

½–1 teaspoon cinnamon

3–4 ice cubes (optional)

1. Place all of the ingredients into a blender and whirl on high until well blended. Chia seeds tend to thicken as they rest, so pour the smoothie into four glasses and serve immediately.

Delicious Protein-Packed Strawberry-Blueberry-Tofu Smoothie

I served this smoothie to friends who are not gluten-free, dairy-free, or vegetarian, and they loved it. You can doctor this recipe up if you want, adding kale, sprouts, chia seeds, or flax seeds, but you may want to keep it simple if you want your kids to drink it. Even this simple recipe is packed with good protein and complex carbohydrates.

MAKES FOUR 8-OUNCE SERVINGS • PREP TIME: LESS THAN 5 MINUTES

1 ripe banana

¼ cup honey or maple syrup (reduce the amount if you want less sweetener)

1 cup coconut, hemp, soy, or almond milk, or milk of your choice

¼ cup organic freshly squeezed orange juice

¾ cup frozen or fresh strawberries (if using fresh berries, add 3–4 ice cubes)

½ cup organic blueberries

12 ounces tofu

½–¾ teaspoon ground cinnamon

1. Mash the banana together with the honey and then put it in a blender. Add the rest of the ingredients and purée until smooth and creamy. If you are using fresh berries, you will need to add 3–4 ice cubes to the smoothie and blend. Pour into four glasses and serve immediately.

Fresh Carrot, Orange, and Avocado Juice

I have a juicer in the house, so I make my own carrot juice. If you don't have a juicer, you can buy organic carrot juice at the market. Drinking this juice is a great way to start the day; to add protein, toss in some chia seeds.

MAKES THREE 8-OUNCE SERVINGS ◆ **PREP TIME: 5 MINUTES**

2 cups fresh carrot juice

1 cup freshly squeezed orange juice

1 ripe avocado

¼ cup fresh parsley

Pinch of cayenne pepper

1. Put all of the ingredients in the blender and whirl until fully blended. Pour the juice over ice cubes in three small glasses and serve.

Slow Cooker Sauce

When I was developing this recipe—with the goal of coming up with an easy and no-fuss but tasty sauce—I threw all of the ingredients in the slow cooker, turned it on high, and estimated it would be done in about 2 hours. I ended up running out to babysit my granddaughter and forgot to turn it off before I left the house. Instead of 2 hours, the sauce cooked for 5 hours! I was worried that I had ruined it, but to my surprise, it was delicious. It has a unique texture and taste, and in addition to eating it on a GF buns (like for Sloppy Junes, page 93), it's great on pasta, polenta, brown rice noodles, spaghetti squash, or quinoa, or as a pizza sauce.

MAKES ABOUT 2 QUARTS • PREP TIME: ABOUT 5 HOURS

1 tablespoon olive oil

1 (12-ounce) package vegetarian chorizo

1 (15-ounce) can organic tomato sauce

1 (6-ounce) can organic tomato paste

1 (28-ounce) can organic crushed tomatoes in sauce

¾ cup water

⅓ cup red wine

1 cup finely chopped onion

1 heaping teaspoon minced garlic (use 2–3 cloves)

3 bay leaves

1 teaspoon fresh tarragon (optional)

¼ cup torn or chopped fresh basil, or more if desired

½ cup chopped fresh parsley

¼–½ teaspoon fresh cracked pepper

½ teaspoon kosher salt

1. Heat a skillet over high or medium-high heat and add the olive oil.

2. When the oil is hot, squeeze out the chorizo from the casing it comes in into the pan. Stir frequently, to avoid sticking, for about 5 minutes, then put it in the slow cooker.

3. Place all the rest of the ingredients into the slow cooker and stir them well. Cover the slow cooker and turn it to high heat.

4. Let the sauce cook for up to 5 hours. If you are going to be away all day and you can't turn it off in 5 hours, set the dial to low and let it cook for 7–8 hours.

5. This recipe makes about 2 quarts of sauce. This sauce can be used in several ways, as mentioned in the headnote, so you will want to store it in an airtight container in the fridge for future use. It will store for up to a week. If you prefer to freeze it, you can split the sauce in half, use some right away and freeze the rest in a storage container.

Note: This recipe calls for vegetarian chorizo (I recommend Helen's Kitchen brand), which is a bit spicy. If you don't like spice or have finicky kids in the house, you might want to use a vegan meat alternative that is not spicy.

Non-Dairy Alfredo Sauce

I have made mock Alfredo sauces in the past using tofu and white beans as the base, but for this recipe, I ventured out of the box and used a nut base. You can find macadamia nuts at most grocery stores, at Trader Joe's, or at your local health-food store. Make sure the nuts are raw and unsalted. I don't recommend substituting other nuts in this recipe because the flavor would not be the same. Macadamia nuts provide a smooth, creamy, buttery flavor. Serve this sauce over brown rice noodles or spaghetti squash noodles.

SERVES 4 ◆ **PREP TIME: ABOUT 5 MINUTES**

2 cups raw unsalted macadamia nuts

1 cup cashew milk (page 198) or store-bought nut milk (such as almond)

3 tablespoons chopped green onions/scallions

1 teaspoon chopped garlic

½ teaspoon sea salt

½ teaspoon nutmeg

2 tablespoons Mock Parmesan Cheese (page 201)

2 tablespoons nutritional yeast

Sea salt and fresh cracked pepper to taste

1. Pulse the macadamia nuts in a food processor (or blender) until the consistency is like a fine meal. Add the rest of the ingredients to the food processor (except the salt and pepper) and whirl until the mixture is creamy and smooth and all of the ingredients are fully incorporated.

2. Remove from the food processor and season with salt and pepper to taste. Serve the sauce over your preferred noodles. Garnish the dish with additional cheese, if desired. Store any leftovers in an airtight container in the fridge for 2–3 days.

Cilantro Pesto Sauce

Pesto can be eaten on brown rice noodles, kelp noodles, or spaghetti squash, or as a spread on your favorite toasted bread, or as a topping for yams or pizza—and more! If you have an allergy to nuts, omit the cashews, and it will still taste great.

MAKES ABOUT 1 CUP • PREP TIME: 10 MINUTES

½ cup chopped raw cashews

1 clove garlic, minced

⅓ cup olive oil

1–2 limes, juiced

1 large bunch fresh cilantro, de-stemmed and washed well

2–3 tablespoons grated Parmesan cheese or Mock Parmesan Cheese (page 201)

Sea salt and fresh cracked pepper to taste

1. Toast the cashews and garlic in a small non-stick skillet over medium heat for about 1–2 minutes, or until the nuts are lightly toasted and the aroma fills your nose. Remove them from the heat.

2. Place the nuts and garlic in a food processor (or blender) and pulse until fine. Add in the olive oil and lime juice and pulse until well blended, then add the cilantro and cheese and continue to pulse until the mixture is very smooth.

3. Season with salt and pepper to taste and serve or store for later. The pesto can be stored in an airtight container in the refrigerator until ready to use. This sauce will stay fresh in the refrigerator for up to a week.

Vegan Hollandaise Sauce

I took this sauce to a party with some grilled vegetables, and everyone loved it! You can store this in the fridge in an airtight container and pull it out to eat with potatoes, quinoa burgers, squash, or grilled veggies (such as asparagus, cauliflower, broccoli, or spinach).

MAKES 2 CUPS ◆ **PREP TIME: 10 MINUTES**

1 cup (8 ounces) organic firm tofu

2 tablespoons nutritional yeast

¼ cup lemon juice, freshly squeezed if possible

2 tablespoons water

1 tablespoon white wine or water

1 teaspoon sea salt

¼ heaping teaspoon turmeric

¼ teaspoon cayenne pepper

4 tablespoons grapeseed oil

Additional sea salt and fresh cracked pepper to taste

1. Break the tofu into chunks and place them in a steamer. Turn the heat to high and steam for 5–6 minutes.

2. Put all of the ingredients into a food processor (except the additional salt and pepper) and pulse until the mixture is smooth and creamy. If you'd like the sauce to be thinner, add more water, wine, or lemon juice. Play around with the texture until the consistency is right for you. Season the sauce with additional salt and pepper, if desired.

Sesame Tahini and Lime Dressing

This dressing is great on a green salad, but I also like to drizzle it over roasted veggies or baked garnet yams. It is also used as the dressing for the Broccoli Salad found on page 67.

MAKES 1 CUP • PREP TIME: LESS THAN 10 MINUTES

3 teaspoons Dijon mustard

3 tablespoons sesame tahini

3 tablespoons coconut cream (or canned coconut milk, full fat)

3 tablespoons grapeseed oil

¼ cup freshly squeezed lime juice

2 teaspoons kelp granules (optional)

¾ teaspoon sea salt

Fresh cracked pepper to taste

1. Place all of the ingredients into a blender or food processor and whirl to fully incorporate. Season to taste with salt and fresh cracked pepper. Store the dressing in an airtight container in the refrigerator.

Almond Curry Dressing

This dressing is delicious tossed with a green salad, used in a kale slaw, or served as a dip for veggies (keep the dip thick by using less water). I kept the seasoning on the light side for this recipe, to appease the kids out there, but add more curry if you want a stronger flavor. Use fresh ginger rather than dried in this recipe, if you happen to have it in the house.

MAKES 1½ CUPS ◆ PREP TIME: 10 MINUTES

¾ cup raw almonds

⅔ cups warm water

2 tablespoons plus 1 teaspoon apple cider vinegar

1½ tablespoons honey or brown rice syrup

1 tablespoon olive oil

¼ teaspoon minced garlic

½ teaspoon Dijon mustard

Pinch of dried ginger (up to ¼ teaspoon)

Pinch of curry (up to ¼ teaspoon)

½ teaspoon sea salt

Fresh cracked pepper to taste

1. Put the almonds in a food processor or a high-speed blender and whirl on full speed for 1–2 minutes, or until they are the consistency of meal.

2. Add the rest of the ingredients and whirl until completely blended. Use immediately or pour into a quart-size glass container and store in the refrigerator. The dressing will keep for several weeks.

3. This dressing thickens over time, so you may need to thin it with water after it has been sitting in the fridge.

Traditional Sauerkraut with a Twist

This is the BEST sauerkraut recipe! Sauerkraut can be used in many different and unusual ways: I put sauerkraut in stir-fried veggies, soups, and breakfast scrambles, and on pizza! It is good for digestion and adds a unique flavor to your dishes. This recipe makes a lot of sauerkraut, so share it or put it into jars and store it in the refrigerator. Sauerkraut is already fermented, so it will store well for up to a month in the refrigerator.

MAKES ABOUT 2 QUARTS • PREP TIME: 1 HOUR, PLUS 10–14 DAYS FOR FERMENTING

4 pounds green cabbage, chopped fine (about 15–16 cups)

2 organic tart apples, peeled and grated (about 2 cups)

2 large organic carrots, peeled and grated (about 2 cups)

1 tablespoon juniper berries

3 tablespoons kosher salt

1. Wash a 1-gallon sauerkraut crock to prepare it for the fermentation process. Working with clean equipment is critical to the process.

2. Prepare the cabbage and set it aside. Place the apple, carrot, and juniper berries into the crock.

3. Add about half of the chopped cabbage (about 6–7 cups) to the crock and sprinkle 1½ tablespoons of the salt over the top. Knead the mixture together for several minutes. I knead the mixture with clean hands (you can use a potato masher if you prefer). Grab and squeeze the mixture aggressively for about 4-5 minutes, until the brine begins to release.

4. Add the other half of the cabbage to the crock with the rest of the salt and knead well, until the brine is released and the cabbage mixture is fully submerged under the brine. The cabbage mixture must be covered with the brine; if it is not, you must do some more massaging, kneading, or punching down of the vegetable mixture with your fist, until it is fully covered with the brine.

Note: You will need a 1-gallon stoneware crock to make this recipe. These can be purchased online at Amazon or at your local hardware store, as can crock weights.

5. Set a crock weight on top of the cabbage mixture in the crock. If you don't have a crock weight, use a plate with full glass of water on top of it to weight it down. Cover the crock with a cheesecloth and place it on a counter at room temperature (65–75°F).

6. In about 6 hours, check the crock to make sure the cabbage is still covered with the brine. If it is, then leave it as is for a couple days. If the cabbage is not covered, then do some more kneading or massaging to create more brine. Put the cheesecloth back on top and then leave it for a couple days.

7. Check the crock again in two days to ensure the brine is still covering the cabbage. If at any time the cabbage is not submerged, simply mash the cabbage down to release more brine. Keep the crock covered with the cheesecloth and allow the cabbage sit for 10–14 days. No need to stir it or check on it after the second day, unless you are worried it isn't submerged under the brine. You can eat it right away, or store it in an airtight container in the refrigerator.

Indian-Style Sauerkraut

Traditionally, sauerkraut is spiced with juniper berries (see the recipe on page 188), but many people replace the berries with other spices, depending on what they like and have available. In this version, I decided to go with an East Indian flavor. The key to great sauerkraut is to really work and knead the cabbage to create a brine that it ferments in for several days or weeks. Some people believe you need to let the fermenting process go much longer than a few weeks, but I am as excited as a child on Christmas morning, so two weeks is the longest I can wait! Feel free to experiment with this recipe and add different spices to create something fun that incorporates your favorite flavors.

MAKES 1½–2 QUARTS • PREP TIME: 1 HOUR, PLUS 10–14 DAYS FOR FERMENTING

2 heads cabbage (about 3–3½ pounds)

1 small onion, minced

4 cloves garlic, minced

2 cardamom pods (optional)

1 teaspoon coriander seeds

1 teaspoon fennel seeds

2 teaspoons cumin seeds

½ teaspoon fresh cracked pepper

2½–3 tablespoons kosher salt

1. Wash a 1-gallon sauerkraut crock to prepare it for the fermentation process. Working with clean equipment is critical to the process.

2. To prepare the sauerkraut, chop all of the cabbage finely and place it in a large bowl. Add the minced onion and garlic, cardamom, coriander, fennel, cumin, and fresh cracked pepper to the cabbage.

3. Put half of the cabbage mixture into a large sauerkraut crock and sprinkle 1½ tablespoons of the salt over the top. With clean hands (or potato masher), knead the cabbage mixture for several minutes. This will help to create the brine that the cabbage will ferment in. It is critical that you keep massaging or kneading (mashing) the cabbage until it begins to release its liquid, about 4–5 minutes.

4. Add the rest of the cabbage mixture to the crock and sprinkle the rest of the salt over the top. Continue to knead well until the brine is released and the cabbage mixture is fully submerged under the brine. If it's not fully submerged, do some more massaging, kneading, or punching down of the vegetable mixture with your fist, until the cabbage is fully covered with the brine.

5. Set a crock weight on top of the cabbage mixture in the crock. If you don't have a crock weight, use a plate with a full glass of water on top of it to weight it down. Cover the crock with a cheesecloth and place it on a counter at room temperature (65–75°F).

6. In about 6 hours, check to make sure the cabbage is still covered with the brine. If it is not covered, do some more kneading or massaging to release more brine. When the cabbage is submerged in brine once again, re-cover the crock with the cheesecloth and leave it for a couple days.

7. Check the crock again in two days to ensure the brine is still covering the cabbage. If at any time the cabbage is not covered in the brine, simply mash the cabbage down. Keep the crock covered with the cheesecloth and let the mixture sit for 10–14 days. No need to stir it or check on it after the second day, unless you are worried the cabbage isn't submerged in the brine. If the smell of the sauerkraut is too much for you, place a secure lid on top of the crock. You can eat it right away, or store it in an airtight container in the refrigerator for up to a month.

Note: Please see details about the type of crock and crock weight to use in the Traditional Sauerkraut recipe on page 188.

Homemade Mushroom Stock

Mushroom stock adds a rich flavor to recipes. I love to use it in hearty soups or in the Mock French Onion Soup with Mushrooms (page 50). Mushroom stock can be difficult to find in your local market, so here is my homemade version. You can store it for up to five days in the fridge in an airtight container, or freeze it in a container for later.

MAKES ABOUT 6 CUPS • PREP TIME: 1–2 HOURS

1 tablespoon coconut oil

1 medium onion, peeled and quartered

6 stalks celery, washed and cut into quarters

1 pound mushrooms, cleaned and de-stemmed

1 tablespoon sun-dried tomatoes, drained

4 cloves garlic

1 tablespoon Bragg's Liquid Amino Acids

6 cups water

½ teaspoon sea salt or kosher salt

Fresh cracked pepper to taste

1 teaspoon fresh thyme (or ½ teaspoon dried thyme)

1. Heat a large stock pot over medium-high heat and add the oil.

2. When the oil is hot, add the onion, celery, mushrooms, and sun-dried tomatoes and sauté for 3–4 minutes, allowing the vegetables to release their flavors. Add the garlic and stir.

3. Reduce the heat to medium and add the Bragg's, water, and seasonings. Simmer for an hour, or longer for a stronger broth.

4. Strain the vegetables from the broth and discard them. Use the stock immediately in a recipe, or store it in an airtight container in the refrigerator or freezer.

Homemade Vegetable Stock

I have experimented with many different vegetable stocks over the years, and I have found that it is important to stick to basic vegetables, such as onions, garlic, carrots, celery, and mushrooms, rather than using fancier vegetables. This stock will keep in the refrigerator for up to five days, but I strongly encourage you to freeze some so you can pull it out when you're in a pinch!

MAKES 7½ CUPS • PREP TIME: 1–2 HOURS

1 tablespoon coconut oil or olive oil

8 stalks celery, washed, ends cut off, and cut into quarters

1 large onion, peeled and quartered

1 (8-ounce) package cremini mushrooms, cleaned and de-stemmed

2 large carrots (about 2 cups chopped)

5 cloves garlic, peeled

9 cups water

1 tablespoon yellow miso

1 tablespoon Bragg's Liquid Amino Acids

2 large bay leaves

25 peppercorns

Pinch of red pepper flakes (optional)

1. Heat the oil in a large stock pot over medium heat.

2. Add in the vegetables and the garlic and sauté for 4–5 minutes, to release the flavors.

3. Add the water, miso, Bragg's, bay leaves, peppercorns, and red pepper flakes and stir to combine. Reduce the heat to medium-low. Simmer the stock for an hour, or longer for a stronger flavor.

4. Strain the vegetables from the broth and discard them. Use the stock immediately in a recipe, or store it in an airtight container in the refrigerator or freezer.

Roasted Almonds

I like to have roasted almonds on hand to use for a quick snack or in various recipes. Toss some roasted almonds in your green salads or use them to make your own almond butter or almond meal.

MAKES 3½ CUPS • **PREP TIME: 12–15 MINUTES**

1 pound raw almonds (about 3½ cups)

1. Preheat the oven to 375°F.

2. Spread the almonds on a baking sheet; I use a clay baking sheet, and the almonds roast very evenly on it. Put the almonds in the oven and roast them for about 12 minutes, stirring once halfway through the bake time. When the nuts are slightly darker in color, remove them from the oven and cool them completely. Store the cooled roasted almonds in an airtight container in the refrigerator so they do not get rancid.

Almond Meal

I use almond meal or flour in a lot of my recipes, but it can be expensive to buy, so I decided to make my own! For about $5.50, I can make about 3½ cups of almond meal. Most of my baked-goods recipes require ½–1 cup almond meal, so this batch will be enough for several recipes.

MAKES ABOUT 3½ CUPS ◆ PREP TIME: 5 MINUTES

1 pound raw almonds (about 3½ cups)

1. Preheat the oven to 375°F.

2. Spread the almonds on a baking sheet; I use a clay baking sheet, and the almonds roast very evenly on it. Put the almonds in the oven and roast them for about 12 minutes, stirring once halfway through the baking time. When the nuts are slightly darker in color, remove them from the oven. Let the almonds cool completely.

3. Place all of the cooled almonds in a food processor equipped with a standard blade and run (do not pulse) until the nuts are finely ground, about 3–4 minutes.

4. Store the almond meal in an airtight container in the refrigerator for use in cookies, cakes, breads, and bars. This meal will store well in the refrigerator in an airtight container for a few months.

Almond Butter

I like making staples like nut butters from scratch, and it's a fun project to do with kids. This smooth and creamy almond butter is super easy to make. It's delicious in sandwiches or cookies, spread onto celery or apple slices, and as a topping for my Delightful Teff Waffles (page 21).

MAKES ABOUT 2 CUPS ◆ PREP TIME: 30 MINUTES

1 pound raw almonds (about 3½ cups)

1 teaspoon kosher salt

1. Preheat the oven to 375°F.

2. Spread the almonds on a baking sheet; I use a clay baking sheet, and the almonds roast very evenly on it. Place the almonds in the oven and roast them for about 12 minutes, stirring once halfway through the baking time. When the nuts are slightly darker in color, remove them from the oven. Let the almonds cool slightly.

3. Place all of the slightly cooled (but not cold) almonds in a food processor equipped with a standard blade and turn on. Do not pulse, just run for about 4–5 minutes, until the almonds are the consistency of meal.

4. Add the salt to the mixture, then pulse to fully incorporate.

5. Separate the mixture into two even batches. Place one batch of the mixture into a bowl and set it aside.

6. With half of the meal in the food processor, turn it on and watch as the almond meal begins to turn to butter. Keep running the food processor until the mixture is smooth and creamy, about 6–7 minutes. Remove the butter from the food processor (make sure to scrape it off the sides) and place it in a quart-size container.

7. Add the rest of the almond meal to the food processor and repeat step 6. Scrape the butter out of the food processor and add it to the container.

8. Store the almond butter in an airtight container in the refrigerator. It will store well for two months or more.

Sunflower Seed Butter

If you or one of your family members are nut-free, sunflower seed butter is a great alternative to almond, cashew, or peanut butter. This recipe takes less than 10 minutes to prepare in your food processor. Use this delicious butter on toast, in cookies, or on celery or apple slices.

MAKES ABOUT ½ CUP ◆ PREP TIME: 12–15 MINUTES

1 cup roasted, unsalted sunflower seeds (organic preferred)

½ teaspoon grapeseed oil (optional)

Sea salt, if desired

1. Place all of the seeds into a food processor equipped with a standard blade. Run the processor (do not pulse) until the seeds turn to the consistency of meal (the amount of time depends on the strength of your food processor but usually a few minutes will do). Turn off the food processor and stir the mixture, scraping down the sides of the bowl.

2. Turn the food processor back on and continue to let it run until the mixture begins to turn into a smooth butter. I recommend stopping it and stirring the mixture at least two or three times. If the butter is too thick, add the grapeseed oil. When you do so, add the oil as the food processor is running so the oil is absorbed into the butter.

3. When the butter reaches the right consistency, usually after 7–9 minutes total, move it from the food processor into an airtight container and season with the salt. Store the butter in the refrigerator and it will last several weeks.

Note: This recipe only makes a small amount of butter, so if you want to make more, do it in two separate batches. If you double the recipe and add twice the amount of seeds into the food processor all at once, the motor will likely burn out. Instead only put 1 cup of the seeds into the food processor at a time!

Cashew Milk

When making cashew milk, you can soak the cashews for a few hours to make them easier to digest, but you don't have to. Soaking is not required because cashews are a soft nut and have no outer skin. Also, because there are no skins, you don't have to strain the milk through cheesecloth. However, if you wish to have extra smooth milk, you can strain it if you'd like.

MAKES 4 CUPS • PREP TIME: LESS THAN 5 MINUTES, PLUS 4 HOURS OPTIONAL SOAKING TIME

4 cups purified water

1 cup raw cashews (soaked in water for up to 4 hours, if desired)

1 tablespoon organic maple syrup

Vanilla extract (optional)

1. Put the water and cashews in a blender and whirl on high for about a minute. The milk will be frothy. Add the maple syrup and vanilla extract and whirl to fully incorporate the ingredients.

2. Strain through cheesecloth, if desired. Store in an airtight container in the refrigerator. Cashew milk will keep for 4–5 days.

Coconut Milk Three Ways

Store-bought milks can be expensive, and they tend to be full of additives. That's why I make my own almond, cashew, and coconut milk. Coconut milk is fun to make, and the results are worth the effort! It is not easy to make milk from raw coconuts, so I have provided three different recipes for homemade coconut milk—choose the one that best fits your time constraints and taste buds.

Version 1: From Whole Raw Coconuts

MAKES 4–5 CUPS ◆ PREP TIME: 10–15 MINUTES

2 whole coconuts

4 cups warm water

1. Crack open the coconuts. Remove the nut from the shell and peel and wash the coconut meat. Retain the coconut water to drink or use in a different recipe.

2. Put the coconut meat with the water into a blender or food processor. Blend or pulse this mixture well, until it is white and frothy.

3. The liquid will be thick, so you will need to strain it. Place 3–4 layers of cheesecloth over a bowl and pour the mixture through. Squeeze the cheesecloth to get all of the milk out of the pulp. Store the milk in an airtight container in the refrigerator, where it will last for a few days. If the fat and liquid begin to separate, shake it up well before using.

Version 2: From Canned Coconut Cream

1. To make coconut milk from canned coconut cream, simply combine one part coconut cream to two parts warm water. Strain the liquid through a cheesecloth so it is not grainy. Store the milk in an airtight container, like a 1-quart jar, in the refrigerator. It will stay fresh for several days.

Version 3: From Shredded Unsweetened Coconut

1½ cups water

7 ounces shredded unsweetened coconut

1. Heat the water in a small saucepan on the stove, but do not bring it to a boil. You want it hot but not boiling.

2. Place the coconut into a food processor with the hot water. Blend for at least 2–3 minutes, or until white and frothy.

3. Pour the milk through 3–4 layers of cheesecloth into a large bowl. Strain the milk a few times, then squeeze the cheesecloth to get all the milk out. Store the milk in an airtight container in the refrigerator. It will last for several days.

Mock Sour Cream

If you are dairy-free or vegan, this alternative for sour cream will be right up your alley! This sour cream is easy to make, stores well in the refrigerator for a week, and tastes refreshing. If you are feeling adventurous, add some fresh chives or dill to the sour cream.

MAKES ABOUT 1 CUP   ◆   PREP TIME: LESS THAN 10 MINUTES

½ cup raw cashews

2 teaspoons yellow miso

¼ cup freshly squeezed lemon juice

¼ teaspoon nutmeg

Sea salt to taste

1. Place the cashews, miso, lemon juice, and nutmeg in a food processor or blender and whirl until the mixture is very smooth and creamy. Season it to taste with salt. Store the sour cream in an airtight container in the refrigerator for up to a week.

Mock Parmesan Cheese (Nut Cheese)

This alternative to soy-based vegan or dairy Parmesan cheese is easy to make, and it has an excellent flavor and is fun to sprinkle over your favorite recipes. It will store well in the refrigerator for several weeks in an airtight container. This is my all-time favorite non-dairy Parmesan cheese!

MAKES: 1 CUP   ◆   PREP TIME: LESS THAN 10 MINUTES

1 cup raw Brazil nuts

1 heaping teaspoon minced fresh garlic (about 2 cloves)

½ teaspoon salt (I like Himalayan salt)

Fresh cracked pepper to taste (optional)

1. Place the Brazil nuts, garlic, and salt into a food processor. Run the food processor for about 30 seconds, or until the mixture is finely ground. Season with fresh cracked pepper to taste, if desired.

Acknowledgments

I would like to thank all of the people who volunteered to sample or make the recipes included in this book, those who provided ideas for recipes, and those who helped in a variety of other ways during this process, such as those who helped at the photo shoot or did the proofreading. There are so many to thank, I apologize if I have left anyone out. These folks really stepped up to the plate to lend a hand, and I am grateful for their feedback and contributions to the book. Thank you to Barb Schiltz, Sally Johnson and family, and the staff at Ocean-fit Yoga Studio (especially Billy, Laura, and Tina). I also want to thank CC Chapman, Wayne Cliffe, Christine and Ryan Shaw, Joe and Lucy Leicht, Dave Barlet, Jessie Bjorklund, Rory Berthiaume, Stephanie Ann, Shay McDonnell, Dr. Casia Coppola, Lila Coppola, Enzo Coppola, Randy and Logan Norton, L. Wheeler, Noralee Sherman, Nadine, Chuck Lowrey, Kay Rusoff, Will Johnson, Paul Dragg and Nanci Stahlman, Keith Yoshida, Jerry Weeks, Marcia Doran, Karin Hawn, Sheila Jantzen, Annie Proctor and all of the folks who attended the first-ever GF October Fest in San Diego, all of the members who taste-tested my recipes at the San Clemente Community Market/Co-op, all of my followers on my Facebook page (Gluten Free Vegan), Terry and Marie Tucker, David Weisenthal, and Joan Fredin. I would also like to thank the food stylist, Paula Rivera, and the photographers John and Deb Svoboda and Fidel Malfavon. I also wish to thank my editor at Da Capo Press, Dan Ambrosio, his editorial assistant, Claire Ivett, and project editor Amber Morris, who all truly did an amazing job editing this cookbook.

To my family and close friends who put up with me while I spent hours in the kitchen and refused to come out and play: thank you! I appreciate your unending support. To my best friend, Carol Dudley: your support never wavers, and for that I am eternally grateful.

And to my dad, who loved to cook and bake until he was in his eighties, and who encouraged me to try, try, and try again until I got it right.

Cooking Equivalents and Metric Conversions

COOKING EQUIVALENTS

A pinch or dash		will be slightly less than ⅛ teaspoon
3 teaspoons	=	1 tablespoon
4 tablespoons	=	¼ cup
2 tablespoons	=	1 liquid ounce
1 cup	=	½ pint
4 cups of flour	=	1 pound of flour
2 cups of liquid	=	16 ounces
1 cup of uncooked rice	=	2 cups of cooked rice
1 lemon	=	¼ cup lemon juice
1 teaspoon chia seeds mixed	=	1 egg (replacement) with 2 tablespoons of water

METRIC CONVERSIONS

✓The recipes in this book have not been tested with metric measurements, so some variations might occur. Remember that the weight of dry ingredients varies according to the volume or density factor: 1 cup of flour weighs far less than 1 cup of sugar, and 1 tablespoon doesn't necessarily hold 3 teaspoons.

GENERAL FORMULA FOR METRIC CONVERSION

Ounces to grams	multiply ounces by 28.35
Grams to ounces	multiply ounces by 0.035
Pounds to grams	multiply pounds by 453.5
Pounds to kilograms	multiply pounds by 0.45
Cups to liters	multiply cups by 0.24
Fahrenheit to Celsius	subtract 32 from Fahrenheit temperature, multiply by 5, divide by 9
Celsius to Fahrenheit	multiply Celsius temperature by 9, divide by 5, add 32

OVEN TEMPERATURE EQUIVALENTS

FAHRENHEIT (F) AND CELSIUS (C)

100°F	=	38°C
200°F	=	95°C
250°F	=	120°C
300°F	=	150°C
350°F	=	180°C
400°F	=	205°C
450°F	=	230°C

LINEAR MEASUREMENTS

½ inch	=	1½ cm
1 inch	=	2½ cm
6 inches	=	15 cm
8 inches	=	20 cm
10 inches	=	25 cm
12 inches	=	30 cm
20 inches	=	50 cm

WEIGHT (MASS) MEASUREMENTS

1 ounce	=	30 grams		
2 ounces	=	55 grams		
3 ounces	=	85 grams		
4 ounces	=	¼ pound	=	125 grams
8 ounces	=	½ pound	=	240 grams
12 ounces	=	¾ pound	=	375 grams
16 ounces	=	1 pound	=	454 grams

VOLUME (DRY) MEASUREMENTS

¼ teaspoon	=	1 milliliter
½ teaspoon	=	2 milliliters
¾ teaspoon	=	4 milliliters
1 teaspoon	=	5 milliliters
1 tablespoon	=	15 milliliters
¼ cup	=	59 milliliters
⅓ cup	=	79 milliliters
½ cup	=	118 milliliters
⅔ cup	=	158 milliliters
¾ cup	=	177 milliliters
1 cup	=	225 milliliters
4 cups or 1 quart	=	1 liter
½ gallon	=	2 liters
1 gallon	=	4 liters

VOLUME (LIQUID) MEASUREMENTS

1 teaspoon	=	⅙ fluid ounce	=	5 milliliters
1 tablespoon	=	½ fluid ounce	=	15 milliliters
2 tablespoons	=	1 fluid ounce	=	30 milliliters
¼ cup	=	2 fluid ounces	=	60 milliliters
⅓ cup	=	2⅔ fluid ounces	=	79 milliliters
½ cup	=	4 fluid ounces	=	118 milliliters
1 cup or ½ pint	=	8 fluid ounces	=	250 milliliters
2 cups or 1 pint	=	16 fluid ounces	=	500 milliliters
4 cups or 1 quart	=	32 fluid ounces	=	1,000 milliliters
1 gallon	=	4 liters		

Resources

Bob's Red Mill: www.bobsredmill.com

Celiac Sprue Association: www.celiac.com

The Gluten-Free Mall: www.glutenfreemall.com

National Foundation for Celiac Awareness: www.celiaccentral.org

Living Without: www.livingwithout.com

Gluten-Free Living: www.glutenfreeliving.com

Lundberg Family Farms: www.lundberg.com

The Vegan Society: www.vegansociety.com /lifestyle/food/recipes/gluten-free

Vegiac.com: www.vegiac.com

Vegetarian Times: www.vegetariantimes.com /recipe/gluten-free

For More Information on Organic Foods and GMOs

Mother Jones: www.motherjones.com /environment/2013/08/what-are-gmos-and -why-should-i-care

Center for Food Safety: www.centerforfood safety.org/#

US News & World Report: www.usnews.com /opinion/articles/2013/11/04/dear -washington-voters-genetically-modified -food-should-be-labeled

Non-GMO project: www.nongmoproject.org /learn-more/gmos-and-your-family

Harvard School of Public Health on GMOs: http://chge.med.harvard.edu/topic /genetically-modified-foods

Harvard School of Public Health on Health Implications of GMOs: http://chge.med .harvard.edu/resource/human-health -implications-genetically-modified-crops -excerpt-sustaining-life

For More Information on Sustainable Foods

Sustainable Table: www.sustainabletable .org/568/do-you-have-to-eat-100-local -sustainable-and-organic

National Wildlife Federation: www.nwf.org /Eco-Schools-USA/Become-an-Eco -School/Pathways/Sustainable-Food/Tips .aspx

Michael Pollan, Author of *Cooked*: http:// michaelpollan.com/resources

Local Harvest: www.localharvest.org

Buy From the Farm: http://buyfromthefarm.ca

USDA Farmers Markets List: www.ams.usda
.gov/AMSv1.0/farmersmarkets

Organic Consumers Association: www.organic
consumers.org

Slow Food USA: www.slowfoodusa.org

Cooperative Grocer Network: www.cooperative
grocer.coop/coops

Culinate: www.culinate.com/home

Eat Local Challenge: www.eatlocalchallenge
.com

For More Information About the Great Foods Used in this Cookbook

Sprouts: http://sproutpeople.org/sprouts
/nutrition/science; www.care2.com/green
living/10-reasons-to-eat-sprouts.html#
ixzz2uHnSl5yg

Maple Syrup: http://healthnewsreport.blog
spot.com/2011/04/maple-syrups-health
-benefits.html

Honey: www.webmd.com/diet/features
/medicinal-uses-of-honey

Index